C ELI ENOH ELOHIM

The 1ˢᵗ Horn of the Apocalypse Beast

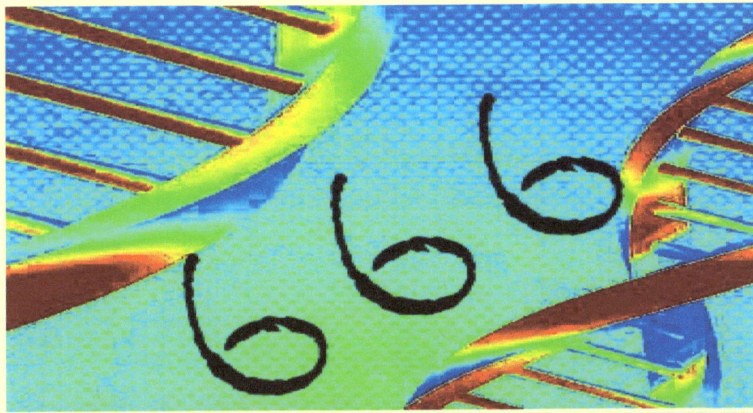

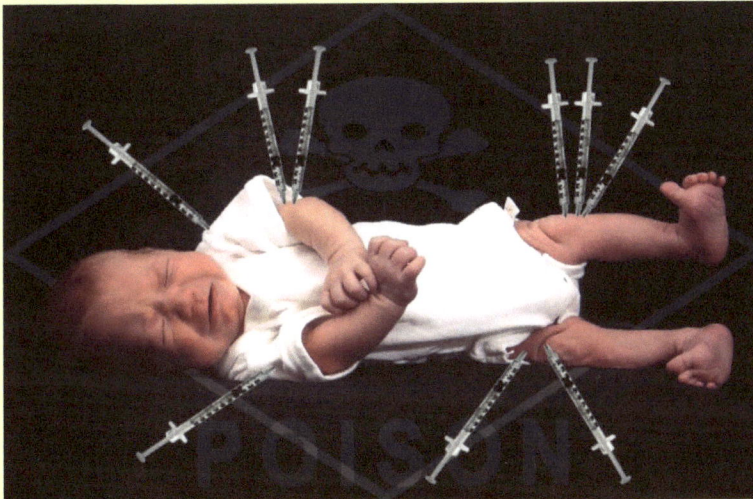

ISBN for PDF e-book : 978-973-0-15921-9

ISBN for printed edition : 978-973-0-15920-2

book two of

The Angel from the 7ᵗʰ Dimension

Published by - **C ELI ENOH ELOHIM** *- Bucharest, 2013*

DEDICATION:

To the terminally ill children without parents from ROMANIA who were deliberately infected with HIV virus in the immunization campaigns after 1989 by Western Europe's vaccines given as *"donation"* to the orphanages...

The informations about HIV infection in Romania in February 1997, were as follows: 3,121 people with HIV and 85% children and 4,446 people with AIDS, of which 4,005 CHILDREN...

Nowadays (in 2013) all the statistical information about this problem are strict classified in Romania by National Health System. The TRUTH is still remaining behind the dust of the top secret files...

Maybe today the deliberately infected innocent orphans are teen-ages, some of them maybe they are young adults and most of them are certainly dead after the AIDS disease-causing them lots of pain in solitude , dying in unhappy hospital conditions, it is good that always to remember them and to try to help the survivors, if exists any of them....

Those Angels have died by a criminal hand... May GOD rest them in peace!

Remark: All the money from selling this book will go as DONATION to the ill children without parents from Romania's orphanages...

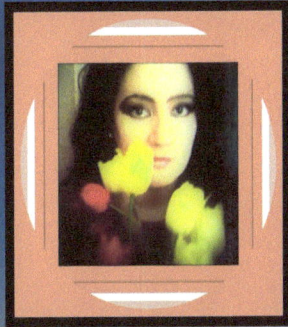

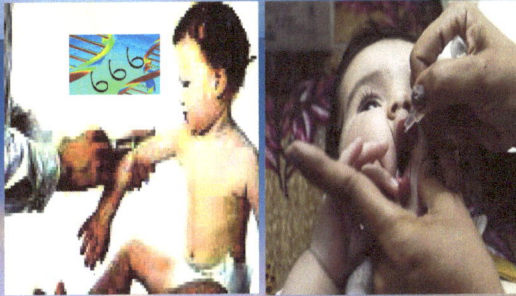

A FEW WORDS ABOUT THE AUTHOR :

C ELI ENOH ELOHIM is the artistic name of Cecilia Spearpoint.

She was born in Romania at 7th May 1968. She has been living her childhood in the shadow of the communist regime and in a conflictual family life. From the childhood she had many prophetic dreams and the ability to see parts of the future that became reality. After she had graduated in 1994 a Technically University in Iassy she became electrical engineer with diploma of licence. She didn't find a job in this field, but she won a mass media competition and she started a job as a journalist in a daily newspaper. She wrote many articles about the social life in Romania.

But... her life has to be different again. Suddenly, in a holiday she became very ill. In 3 days, she lost the ability to walk and she was paralized all body. She has been in a coma 4 weeks and she was in danger to die.

After she received the blessing from the Christian Orthodox Church she begun suddenly to have a very good health. After she learnt to walk again she found out a 72 hours/week job as an electric engineer in a turkish factory from Bucharest. Her life changed again. She was forced to put her resignation after she lost her un-born child in a work accident in the factory. Very soon, she found another job as marketing director and she returned spiritually to the ancient romanian traditional Christian Orthodoxy.

Her life changed again. In 2003, she was about 20 minutes in a clinically death on the street in Bucharest. She came back to life before the ambulance has arrived. After she encountered a Light Angel in her dreams, telling her about prophecies about the future, she decided to became a writer to tell to the world about her experiences.

Mrs Cecilia Spearpoint is married with Adam Spearpoint and they have together a daughter. They are living in England and they have a house in Romania, too. This book has 3 parts and it is inspired by the life of the author and by The Holy Ghost.

C ELI ENOH ELOHIM is a name of a Light Angel who came in a dream to tell to the author of this book prophecies about the future and about the end times...

The Christian Orthodox new prophecies are revealed in the ISBN 978-973-0-15920-2. printed edition

THE ANGEL FROM THE 7th DIMENSION

WW.FACEBOOK.COM / C.ELI.ENOH.ELOHIM

PUBLISHED by C ELI ENOH ELOHIM

Contents:

NOTES ...

The copyright page

Published by **C ELI ENOH ELOHIM**

Romania, Bucharest , 28.12.2013

ISBN for PDF e-book : **978-973-0-15921-9**

ISBN for printed edition : **978-973-0-15920-2**

THE CONTRIBUTORS OF THE BOOKS:

◆ **My mother, Maria GHEORGHIU, who always believed in me;**

◆ **My daughter, Maria D. SPEARPOINT, who was vaccinated with many dangerous and useless vaccines by the GP Doctor L. Chiruta. All of the GP doctors from Romania never gave information to the parents about the poisons from vaccines.**

◆ **The Angel Entity C ELI ENOH ELOHIM who inspired the trilogy   :**

"The Angel from the 7th Dimension".

MOTTO:

"…Than you will know the Truth, and

the Truth will set you free…"

John the Evangelist 8: 32 / The Holy Bible

VERY IMPORTANT WARNING ABOUT THE POISONS FROM THE VACCINES
that are killing the immunity

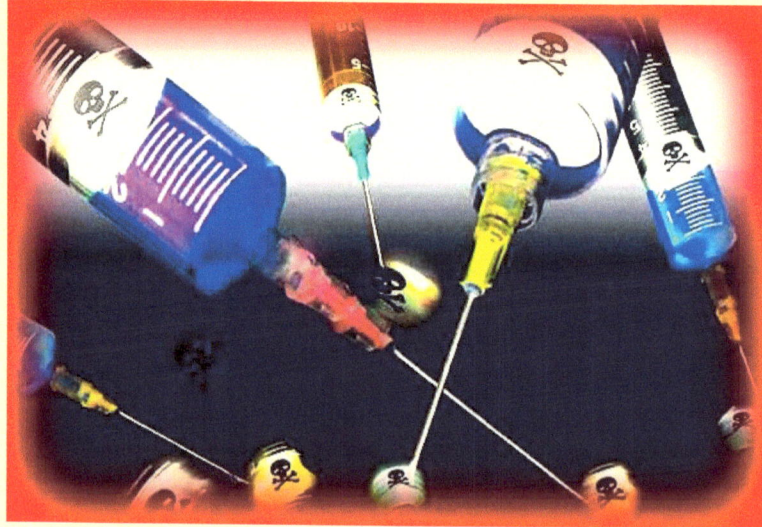

"*These people are against GOD, these people are certainly the servants of **devil**, who hate any creature and divine creation, forgetting that they were all made by the same GOD...But all will collapse...And it has been created a hell in this world, that is struggling them without a way out... So, the powers has unleashed **devil** and now GOD allows the mankind to suffer... However, I do not understand WHY all people are silenced, even valuable people, scientists, intellectuals and they are still living among us and they seem hypnotized by the evil.*"
(Father JUSTIN PARVU – from "The PETRU VODA" Christian Orthodox Monastery , ROMANIA) .

GENERAL INTRODUCTION

In my religious visions I received an information from THE ANGEL FROM THE 7th DIMENSION, that the Evil gave the bad idea of the "immunizations campaigns" to his obedient servants " the malefic scientists"....

So, in the end of the 18th century the first type of "vaccine" was made by stinging a healthy person with a poisoned kind of knife full with the infection to be cured...(!)

If you are an intelligent person and you have an open mind than you will find out that this is a non-sense... How you can make somebody strong by inoculating him an infection directly in the bloodstream?

After more than two centuries of ignorance and manipulation, nowadays most of people are still believing that vaccinations are good...

I will try to show some solid scientific explanations in this book with a lot of medical proofs that :

VACCINES ARE NOT GOOD AT ALL!

However, the medical studies are not exhaustive on this issue, and the hidden truth is evident for the people who really wants to see the truth. Who denies the truth and the evidences, than he does not want to see the truth or maybe he has other interests ...

The vaccinations immunizations campaigns have a specific place even in JOHN' s REVELATION book, because the action of the number of 666 will not exist in the next future, in my opinion, without the mass IMMUNIZATIONS CAMPAIGNS with GENETICALLY

11

MODIFIED VIRUSES IN LABORATORIES.

THE TARGET IS TO MAKE ALL THE PEOPLE OBEDIENT TO THE ANTICHRISTIC SYSTEM THAT IS ALREADY RULLING THE WORLD!

In the next future , after a devastated nuclear war, the 666 ultimatum seal will be an inoculation of a vaccine of a malefic strain of viruses DNA, together with a very sophisticated nanotechnology that will able to guide the malefic DNA to the human brain and put together that "things" there for ever...

I begun to wrote about this important issue in my genuine book : **"THE ANGEL FROM THE 7ᵗʰ DIMENSION ".**

The Christian-Orthodox old priests said that the **666** *hoax will be come a reality only if people will want it so desperately and they will make an oath* **against Christ and against GOD...**

In my opinion, accepting vaccination of your children **after** *you will read this book , it is perfectly equal to be* **against GOD** *and you are friend with devil himself!*

This means that you do not love your children and if you love them why you want to poison them with vaccines?!

If you still accept vaccines that means that you are irresponsible as a parent and you deserve ill children ...(MY REMARK : the majority of the vaccinated children become very ill in their future !)

I have spoken with HUNDRED of people PRO and AGAINST VACCINATION. There were more than 80% of the people who reject vaccines after they got the information and the proofs that vaccines are dangerous poisons. This statistics are available only in Romania and Germany. In USA the vaccines are mandatory.

The most shocking thing is that people who loves vaccines **after** *they got the TRUE information about vaccines ,* **they do** NOT **WANT to change anything in their life**, *because they are born from generation with this idea that vaccines are perfect. This idea will bring lots of pain, illness and* **death** *in their lives!*

I AM NOT SPEAKING ABOUT RICH PEOPLE PAYED TO LIE IN THE MASS MEDIA BECAUSE OF A INTEREST !

I AM SPEAKING ABOUT INTELLIGENT PEOPLES WHO LOVE TRUTH AND WHO REALLY LOVE THEIR CHILDREN!

There is no safe vaccine! **NONE OF THEM ARE GOOD! REJECT ALL VACCINES FROM YOUR LIFE! GIVE A CHANCE TO YOUR CHILDREN :**

SAY NO TO EVERY KIND OF VACCINES!

*The parents who will accept the vaccines for their children **after** they read this book, certainly they DO deserve **ill** children!*

*But if their children will be asked, they will say **NO** to vaccines! The children deserve the right to be healthy, not poisoned with vaccines!*

How an intelligent and responsible parent can give en purpose (deliberately) poison to your child ? You are against GOD and you have to be afraid of GOD!

THE VACCINES OF TODAY ARE INDEED VERY DANGEROUS !

The "INNOCENT" beginning of the number / seal / identification RFID of 666 is the electronic chip , the code bars... But the end is very sophisticated, very dangerous and leads to death in big pains.

*The inoculation of the final **666** seal in the human body will be in the next future only through a vaccination helped by a nanotechnology when the malefic DNA will be sneaking into the brain and killing the person afterwards in very big pain...*

*Maybe less then a decade in the NEXT future, of course that the authorities of the planet (on that time will be only one government ruling all countries after the future devastated WW III). That malefic authority (**BEAST**) will tell big lies to people imposing mandatory vaccination because of a "dangerous epidemic disease".*

The 666 seal will be a triple nucleotides chains , probably this triple chain of DNA (which consists of two chains of human DNA and a strain chain of a STRANGE DNA from something very malefic : viruses or a

13

new life form created in the laboratory) was seen by Jesus Christ apostle John the Evangelist in the REVELATION BOOK.

The 3rd DNA chain will be linked by the other 2 chains by a NANO-CHIP (with a specific bar code – again 666 – a personal number for everybody, no names, only numbers!) who will give perturbations in the human body and death in very big pain.

This implant will never be rejected and the people having the implant will be like zombies – or maybe the perfects slaves, solders – people who will not thinking at all and they will receive information from the BEAST – a person, a big server or devil himself...

This is a nightmare and only a very malefic mind can build this into reality.

The planet is already ruled by a few extremely rich families   (the Bilderberg group , the very rich bankers, the masonry, etc.)- more info on the internet and in mass media), who are controlling everything, including governments, political leaders and all the world 's organizations. They are starting wars all over the planet.

Believe me, the evil in their minds is so high, especially in that families of very rich bankers who are ruling the planet and who are worshipping to Satan, so, they will do their best to have their plans fulfilled. This is not a conspiracy theory, it is already reality.

The prophecies of REVELATION of Saint John the Evangelist is about a great war , vaccinations campaign, the poisoning of water, food and this is for reducing the world population transforming the survivors into their slaves with the 666 seal.

All that people that received the 666 will die with lots of pain and their souls will not be in the heaven.

Who really believes in GOD and JESUS CHRIST, let's pray together and ask for GOD' s Mercy and protection ! Until that biblical times will come true (maybe tomorrow) , make yourself a favour : it is about a n important step against evil .

DO NOT ACCEPT VACCINES IN YOUR LIFE!   IT IS

POISON!

DO NOT ALLOW ANY KIND OF VACCINATION FOR YOUR CHILDREN! SAY NO TO VACCINES!

THE PERPETUATIONS OF THE VACCINES IN THE ALIVE HUMANS BODIES is only by flesh and blood since the end of 18 century when was invented the 1st "vaccine".

Only by immunizations campaigns were preserved the strains of all viruses, most of them would have been disappeared without this devilish invention .

The statistics shown that AFTER the immunizations, the diseases increased and the result was up side down, and authorities and big pharmaceuticals said only lies.

The truth is that vaccines are not efficient, the vaccines do not stop the illness and all the vaccines are very dangerous for the health and kill the immune system of human body.

The evidence is here in this book that it is not addressed to doctors. This book is addressed to the public. So, if there will be any mistake of translation of the medical words I do apologize. I am a scientist and I've graduated a technically university, but I am not a doctor.

However, I read hundreds of books about medicine to be able to understand the medical studies.

A responsible person can find more evidence on the internet and speak with more than 100 doctors. Ask them politely if they are agree with the vaccinations of their own children or grandchildren.

*If the doctors are not afraid of losing their jobs and bonuses, they have to tell you the **HIDDEN TRUTH ABOUT the VACCINES** and about the billions of $, GPB , EURO of the malefic industry of vaccines all over the world .*

If you want more information , you can read my 1st book of the trilogy, which is part one of this book. I have got my own religious *revelations about the end times directly from* <mark>*<THE ANGEL FROM THE 7th DIMENSION>.*</mark>

How I took the decision

to write this book?

About some of the U.K. Doctors...

IT IS A VERY IMPORTANT

PUBLIC HEALTH PROBLEM!

Even it is very dangerous for health, the majority of United Kingdom'"'s GP Doctors recommend VACCINATIONS! Be very careful when you receive the inoculation of the viruses !

The viruses, even attenuated, they are still alive and they do not have the typical side effects and immediate, because the vaccine weakens the immune system of the patient and is vulnerable to surface aspects of the individual's genetic structure.

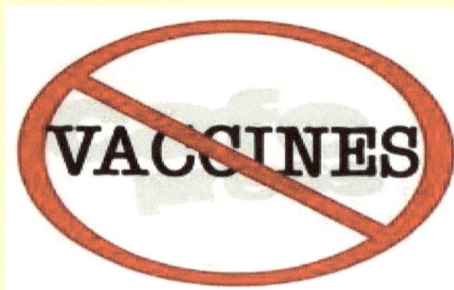

WHY the EVILS' *DOCTORS* DO NOT WANT TO TAKE INTO CONSIDERATION

OTHERS DOCTORS OPPINIONS and RECENTLY MEDICAL REASEARCHES ?

Recently, Dr.N.Payne from BROMLEY South Lodge Surgery, (Kent, Great Britain, U.K.), is not like Mother Theresa, but she is very happy to be obedient to NHS (National Health System). WHY? Because she is very well paid, even her medical training and ability to be a good doctor in medicine is at a very low standards.

Doctor Payne is working a couple of hours a day for a huge salary of more than 100,000 pounds per year. Like lots of doctors in that surgery (the exemption is only Dr. Mary Matthews who is the best of the medical staff) , Doctor Nicola Payne and Doctor Bola Idowu and Doctor Sally Carson are giving the same type of weak and useless antibiotics prescription, after more than two hours waiting at their doors, does not matter what illness you may have.(!) Especially Doctor Idowu is jumping the list of her patients and she is putting the other to wait two hours in front of her door for a non-sense prescription.

Dr B.Idowu and Dr N.Payne are not able to put a diagnostic and are not able to see what illness you or your child may have. They are not good doctors and they care only about their money and contract with NHS. They do not have a strong training into the medicine field, even they like to be called as "doctors"!

Dr.Payne gave me a shocking statement in a <u>ABSOLUTELY CYNIC</u> bad manner: "LEAVE ME ALONE! I do respect you but...I DO "BELIEVE" IN VACCINES. <u>AFTER I</u> HAVE READ ALL THE MEDICAL STUDIES, I DO LIKE THE POISON

17

MERCURY & ALUMINIUM HIDROXIDE FROM VACCINES. I DO NOT
WANT TO READ   OTHER MEDICAL STUDIES OR THOSE HUNDREDS
 OF BOOKS AGAINST VACCINATION WRITTEN BY DOCTORS FROM
GERMANY, USA, ROMANIA, FRANCE. I DO NOT WANT TO FIGHT &
I DO NOT WANT TO OPEN MY MIND! NO MORE MEDICAL STUDIES!
 I DO NOT CARE about DELIBERATELY INFECTED HIV FOUR
THOUSAND ROMANIAN CHILDREN in 1989 by vaccines made in
Western Europe! ".

Doctor Payne is a GP family doctor. Indeed she wants to give
<pain> to all her patients poisoning them with vaccines... She does
not care at all !

DR. PAYNE and her colleagues doctors from Bromley (KENT)
are deliberately poisoning children with the immunizations
campaigns. In fact, the majority of DOCTORS in England are doing
this thing and they have very huge salaries paid by NHS from taxes.

Lots of doctors in UK are not well trained and you need to have a
seat in the hospitals waiting rooms about 3 or 4 hours with a child
with 40 grd. Celsius fever BEFORE a NHS doctor to come to see that
child. In public hospitals children are not on the 1st place in England.

The elders are 1st seen by the doctors in the hospital waiting
room, doesn't matter that the child is with 40 grd. Celsius or in very
big pain. I took a lesson with my 4 years old very ill daughter waiting
4 hours to be seen by a doctor in the Princess Royal Hospital from
Farnborough, near Bromley , KENT, U.K.

In the same time, a granny was seen 3 times in a hour by a
doctor, the granny had a possible broken wrist, but she was not in
pain and no fever. She was happy making a telephone conversation
with somebody...Of course that the doctor was at a very low standard
of medicine, because he was not able to put a diagnostic to my
daughter and the nurses didn't take any blood tests. (April 2011).

The hilarious thing is that most of the patients do not know
about the dangerous poisons from vaccines! NOBODY TOLD
PEOPLE THE TRUTH ABOUT THE POISON FROM VACCINES!

DUE ALL RESPECT for DOCTOR PAYNE and other doctors, GP, from
Bromley South Surgery , I am saying that : It is against GOD and IT
IS AGAINST HUMANITY WHEN A DOCTOR without full sense of

18

responsibility ***STILL WANTS TO RECOMMEND VACCINATIONS AFTER HE KNEW FROM MEDICAL STUDIES THAT VACCINES ARE DANGEROUS!***

In my opinion, the obsolete management of N.H.S. in U.K. , GIVES BIG REWARDS IN MONEY TO THE GP DOCTORS WHEN THEY COME WITH FULL LIST OF VACCINATIONS DONE.

In my opinion, ONLY A RESPONSIBLE DOCTOR <u>***SAYS NO TO VACCINES***</u>***!***

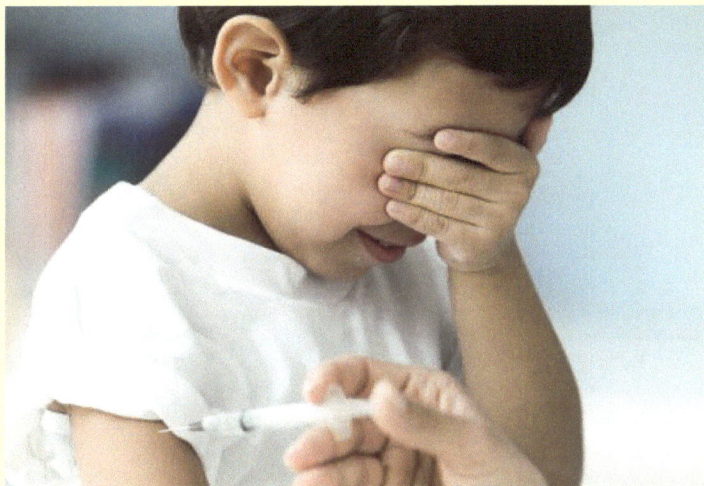

I am polite suggesting that every Doctor who recommends vaccinations, to have himself all "shots" of these poison vaccines and to drink tetra-vaccines, including the rubbish-one "AH1N1", until he will be finished all those 36 vaccines given to a child since birth to 10 years old!

THE POISONS FROM THE VACCINES ARE:

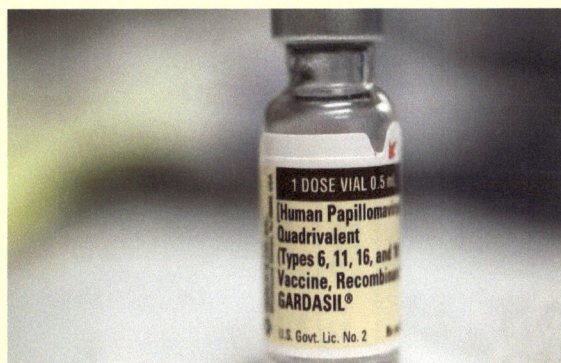

Aluminum Phosphate

Ammonium Sulfate

Casamino Acid

Dimethyl-betacyclodextrin

Formaldehyde

Formalin

Glutaraldehyde

2-Phenoxyethanol

Aluminum Hydroxide,

Bovine Extract

Polysorbate 80.

Aluminum Potassium Sulfate

Thimerosal – MERCURY TOXIC POISON = 50,000 ppb mercury in a "shot" of vaccine and READ below!

Just How Much Mercury?

- .01% solution thimerosal, 0.5 cc dose
- contains 25 mcg of mercury
  - water contamination: 2 ppb
  - toxic waste: 200 ppb
  - fish: 730–1,450 ppb
  - vaccine: 50,000 ppb mercury

Ammonium Sulfate

Lactalbumin Hydrolysate

Monkey Kidney Tissue

Neomycin Sulfate

Polymyxin B

Yeast Protein

Genetically Modified Alive Viruses

(source : http://en.wikipedia.org/wiki/List_of_vaccine_ingredients*)*

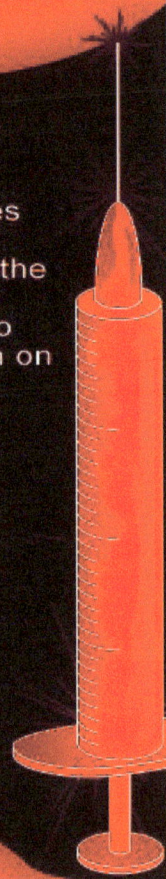

HPV vaccine

Fact:
- Untested
- On the package it states that it does not even prevent cervical cancer
- Even if your school system makes the shot mandatory, you can refuse. No law in the US can force you to take a vaccine. Do your research on the subject or ask a lawyer.

Linked to:
- Loss of Consciousness
- Seizures
- Severe Headaches
- Dizziness
- Temporary Blindness
- Genital Warts
- Permanent Injury
- Paralyzation
- Miscarriages
- Nervous System Damage
- Recurring Painful Rashes
- Death

Keyword Search:
Untested HPV Vaccine

Do you know what's in a vaccine?

Aluminum
Implicated as a cause of brain damage; suspected factor in ALZHEIMER'S DISEASE, dementia, seizures and comas. Allergic can occur on the skin.[1]

Ammonium Sulfate [salt]
Suspected gastrointestinal, liver, nerve and respiratory system POISON.

Beta-Propiolactone
Known to cause CANCER. Suspected gastrointestinal, liver, nerve and respiratory, skin and sense organ POISON.

Gelatin
Produced from selected pieces of calf and cattle skins, de-mineralized cattle bones and pork skin. ALLERGIC reactions have been reported.[1]

Gentamicin Sulfate and Polymyxin B [antibiotics]
ALLERGIC reactions can range from mild to life threatening.[1]

Genetically Modified Yeast, Animal, Bacterial and Viral DNA
Can be incorporated into the recipient's DNA and cause unknown GENETIC MUTATIONS.

Glutaraldehyde
Poisonous if ingested. Causes BIRTH DEFECTS in experimental animals.

Formaldehyde [formalin]
Major constituent of embalming fluid; poisonous if ingested. Probable carcinogen; suspected gastrointestinal, liver, respiratory, immune, nerve and reproductive system POISON.

Human and Animal Cells
Human cells from aborted FETAL TISSUE and human albumin. Pig blood, horse blood, rabbit brain, guinea pig, dog kidney, cow heart, monkey kidney, chick embryo, chicken egg, duck egg, calf serum, sheep blood and others.

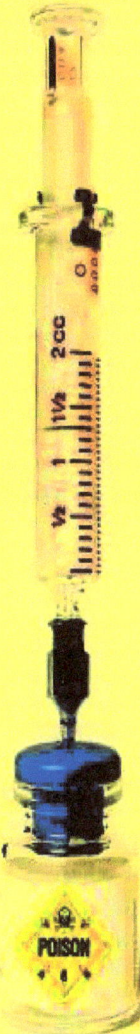

Latex Rubber
Can cause life-threatening allergic reactions.[1]

Mercury [thimerosal]
One of the most poisonous substances known. Has an affinity for the brain, gut, liver, bone marrow and kidneys. Minute amounts can cause nerve damage. Symptoms of mercury toxicity are similar to those of AUTISM.

Micro-Organisms
Dead and alive VIRI AND BACTERIA or their toxins. The polio vaccine was contaminated with a monkey virus, now turning up in human bone, lung-lining (mesothelioma), brain tumors and lymphomas.

Monosodium Glutamate [MSG | glutamate | glutamate acid]
A NEUROTOXIN that's being studied for mutagenic, teratogenic (developmental and monstrosities) and reproductive effects. Allergic reactions can range from mild to severe.[1]

Neomycin Sulfate [antibiotic]
Interferes with vitamin B6 absorption. An error in the uptake of B6 can cause a rare form of epilepsy and mental retardation. ALLERGIC REACTIONS can range from mild to life threatening.[1]

Phenol | Phenoxyethanol [2-PE]
Used as anti-freeze. TOXIC to all cells and capable of disabling the immune system's primary response mechanism.

Polysorbate 80
Know to cause CANCER in animals.

Tri (n) Butylphosphate
Suspected kidney and nerve POISON.

[1] When babies are hours or days old it is impossible to know if they have an allergy.

23

Attention parents !

Any vaccine reduces the immune system

You are the only ones who can refuse!

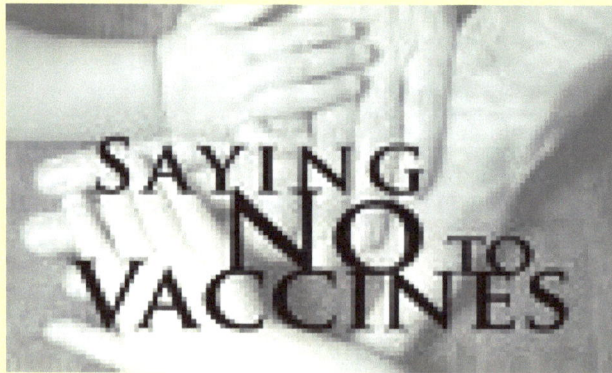

Dr. Buchewald said in the book "The vaccination nonsense": **"The victory against the epidemic was not won by vaccines but the resultant improvements in the technical, social, hygienic and especially nutrition. The hypothesis that vaccines underlying decline of infectious diseases is a great nonsense. "**

Any vaccine is actually a physically assault. Neither doctors nor the authorities tell us that. Any flu shot, wanted or unwanted, including the H1N1 swine flu is actually a physical assault. If I sting you with a needle, you sue me, being a physically assault.

Can you do the same if you are not told about the real risks of the vaccination?

THERE ARE MORE THAN 5,000 PUBLIC SCHOOLS in the U.K. WAITING for TRUE INFORMATION about poisons from vaccines and about others medical problems of the young generations (one example is: do they know that the abortive pills kill for ever the fertility of the young mothers?)

U.K. 's vaccination programmes applies without informing parents about the risks and benefits, often with pressure from doctors, without being informed that the parents are the decision maker, without side effects or consequences to compensate.

In fact, always it has been fed a huge propaganda pro-vaccines by the vaccines producers companies that bribe the officials, the decision makers and sponsors scientific research results, paid PhD scholarships for academics doctors. Who did exactly understand what pseudo-scientific machinery there are "the mandatory vaccines", who thought that the majority of doctors told big lies to cover the dangers of large increasingly diseases for the people exposed?

 Dr. Keisei Gaublomme - *President of International Association "Vaccine Damage Privation*" revealed about the "mechanisms of autoimmune diseases that occur following various vaccinations."

 Dr. Scott Mumby who is a member of the Royal Society of Medicine, a founding member of the British Society for Allergy and nutrition) said that vaccination is a deliberate assault on the developing immune system.

   Health of growing children is weakened by multiple vaccinations introduced by vaccination programmes .

   Dr Shoenefeld realize Immunology (2001) and Tichler (2004) talk about the miserable side of vaccinations. That substances used in the composition of vaccines are: Aluminium, Mercury, triggering THYMEROSAL underlying diseases such as multiple sclerosis, cancer, leukaemia, gastrointestinal severe illnesses.

Vaccines cause the outbreak of autoimmune diseases (diabetes, multiple sclerosis, rheumatic diseases, ulcerative colitis in people genetically predisposed or adversely affect their evolution (sources : Fourni - 2004, Wraith - 2003).

The mobility of genetically material between life forms

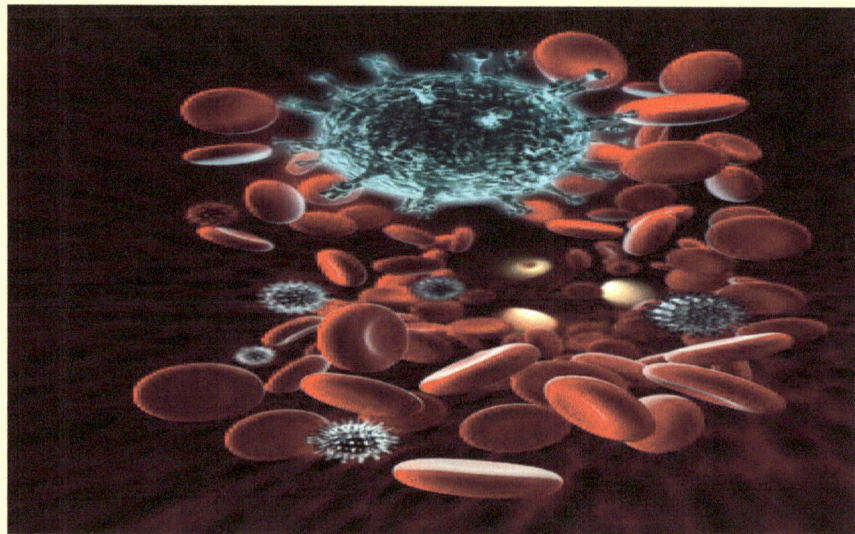

Viruses are among the simplest living organisms, being composed of several strands of DNA or RNA wrapped in a protein capsized spirals.

This extremely simple structure does not allow them to live independently, but only inside a living cell to provide nutrition and reproductive conditions. Currently, there are two major types of cells used in vaccine production: cells of animal (monkey kidney, chick embryo, etc.) & cells of human origin.

The cells of human origin, it is known that, normally, they do not survive outside the human body.

None of the vaccines currently available for any of the diseases is not really effective and it not have been scientifically proven effective vaccines, but on the contrary has been shown that they are very dangerous, sending a large number of viruses.

In addition, substances that are part of vaccines, like mercury and aluminium, can cause <u>autism, leukaemia, Alzheimer disease , cancer,</u>

26

etc.

Since September 1971 became very clear to clever doctors that vaccination is altering the genetic structure of human body.

At that time in Geneva scientists discovered that biological substances entering directly into the bloodstream could become part of the human genetic code. Originally, the Japanese bacteriologists found that bacteria of one species transferred their antibiotic resistance bacteria in a completely different species.

Dr. Maurice and Dr. Philip Anker Stroun from the Department of Plant Physiology at the University of Geneva, began to accumulate evidences that the transfer of genetic information is not limited to bacteria, but can occur and the species from bacteria to higher plants and animals. According to an article in "World Medicine" of September 22, 1971, "Geneva scientists are convinced that animals and plants can release normal DNA and the DNA is taken up by other cells of another organism."

In one experiment, the scientists in Geneva extracted the auricles of frog hearts and dipped them for several hours in a suspension of bacteria.

Then they found a high percentage of DNA-RNA hybridization between bacterial DNA extracted from the same species of bacteria as that used in the experiment and titrated DNA extracted from the auricles which had been immersed in bacterial suspension. Bacterial DNA was absorbed by the animal cells.

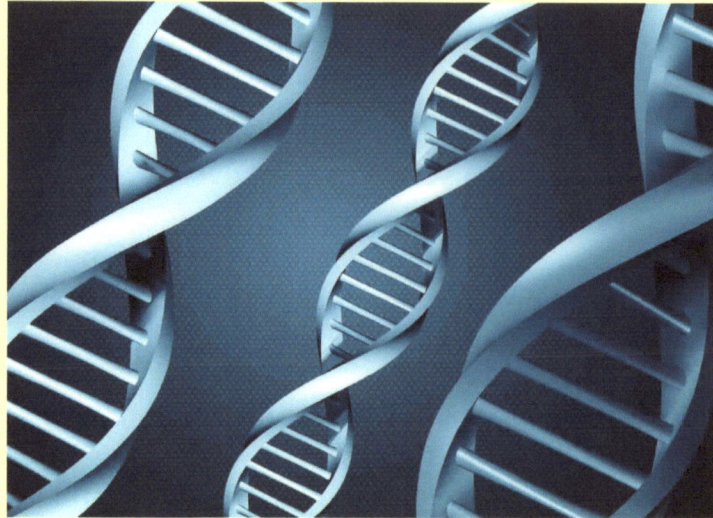

This phenomenon was called "trance-cessions". There is evidence that this phenomenon always occurs inside the human body.

Presumably, such as heart damage following rheumatic fever could be a result of the immune system against its own cells producing a foreign RNA following the absorption of foreign DNA.

In the journal "Science" of November 10, 1972, appeared an article which has been shown in frog brain cells after a bacterial RNA was found peritoneal bacterial infection. In the April 1973 "Journal of Bacteriology" spontaneously released bacterial DNA was found embedded in cell nucleus of frog auricles.

Studies by *Phillipe Anker and Maurice Stroun* production showed the following phenomena: processes of spontaneous release of DNA from mammalian cells, spontaneous transfer of DNA from bacteria to higher organisms, spontaneous transfer of DNA between cells of higher organisms, release of RNA in mammalian cells and biological activity of released complexes containing RNA. Malignant cell transformation caused by foreign DNA.

There is evidence that circulating foreign DNA can cause malignant transformation. In a number of 1977 "International Review of Cytology", Volume 51, Anker and Stroun discuss possible effects of foreign DNA in malignant cell transformation. When foreign DNA is transcribed in a cell of a different body, "this general biological event is related to uptake by cells of spontaneously released bacterial DNA, suggesting the existence of circulating DNA.

Since malignant transformations obtained with DNA, it is postulated role of oncogene (cancer causing) of circulating DNA. "

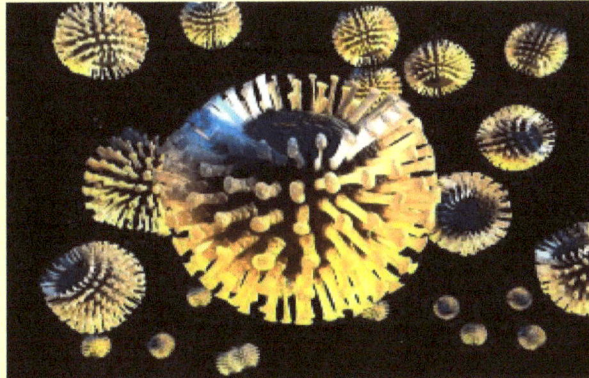

The problem became even more interesting after 1975 when it was discovered that viruses cause cancer in animals possess a special enzyme called reverse transcription. These viruses are called RNA viruses. An RNA virus that possesses reverse transgression in its structure, has the ability to form chains of DNA which easily integrate into the DNA of the host cell that a virus has infected.

Studies by Dr. Robert Simpson of Rutgers University indicate that RNA viruses do not cause cancer can also form DNA, even without the presence of reverse transcription. DNA formed in this way, in an RNA virus is called pro- virus. We know that some viruses tend to persist in cells as pro-virus long time, without cause, apparently, any disease. In other words, remain dormant. Common examples of RNA viruses which cause cancer, but are able to form pro-virus are: influenza (flu), measles, mumps and polio virus. On October 22, 1967 issue of the "British Medical Journal", German researchers have found that MS seems to be caused by vaccinations against smallpox, typhoid, tetanus, polio, tuberculosis and diphtheria. Even earlier, in 1965, the Zintchenko reported 12 cases in which multiple sclerosis occurred after rabies vaccination.

Remember that between 1950-1970, million of people were

injected with polio vaccines (anti-polio) which contained the simian virus 40 (the monkey virus called SV-40), vaccines transferred from contaminated monkey kidney , used to grow the vaccine. It is impossible to remove animal viruses from vaccine cultures. Please remember that SV-40, the 40th simian virus found in tissues is an oncogene virus (causing cancer).

Mass vaccination programs against influenza, measles, mumps and polio, in fact seeding humans with RNA and pro-virus to become latent for long periods inside the human body, and that are activated later in life.

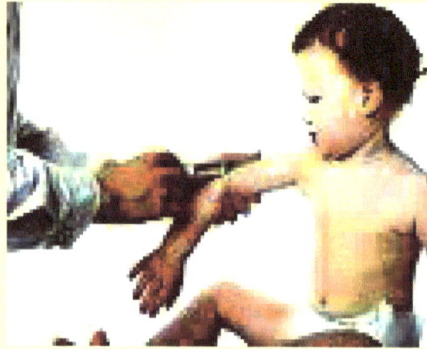

Post-polio syndrome is a good example of this. Other examples may include so-called collagen diseases, rheumatoid arthritis, multiple sclerosis and lupus erythematous.

The immune system produces antibodies against the patient's own tissues - tissues that have been impregnated with foreign genetic material.

According to a special issue of "Postgraduate Medicine" from 1962, "although the human body does not produce under normal conditions, antibodies against its own tissues, it turns out that small changes in the antigenic character of tissues may cause those tissues to be identified as foreign by the immune system and thus become a target for antibody production. "

Two years later, in 1964, studies were made on polyoma virus, a DNA virus maker tumours. Was found that persistent genetic DNA in polyoma virus caused malignant transformation in hamster embryo cell cultures. This discovery was published in the November

23, 1964 the "Journal of the American Medical Association". Even common viruses, non-cancer, including those of smallpox vaccine and polio-virus 2, can act as oncogenes (cancer producing).

In the journal "Science" of 15 December 1961 was reported that these common viruses acted as catalysts in producing cancer when mice were administered in combination with organic substances known carcinogens, the latter being given in amounts too small to cause cancer by themselves.

This means that some vaccinations will induce cancer when combined with the effect of increasing environmental pollution by toxic products of agriculture (pesticides on and in food) and industry.

Of course, this information is hidden from the public for the FDA (Food and Drug Administration), EPA and agriculture-based industries to move forward with the "approval" of small amounts of pollutants in food, water and air.

Contact the pollutants mentioned above has not been disclosed to the delight of the chemical industry, the National Cancer Institute and the industry developed around the cancer, which continues fraudulently, to seek public donations to justify its existence. As an aside, has been recognized that vaccination against polio caused 100% of cases of polio in the U.S. after 1980 and most cases of paralytic poliomyelitis after 1972 ("Science", April 4, 1977). It is suspected that the Salk polio vaccine and Sabin anti-produced by tissue culture of monkey, are also responsible for increased leukaemia in the U.S..

Given that this information is known for over 20 years, the use of viruses, bacteria and animal tissues in mass vaccination campaigns are intentionally creating a risk to human body. Overall impact on the great diversity of the human genotype is difficult to assess, but the impact is undoubtedly negative and allows seeding humans with latent pro-virus.

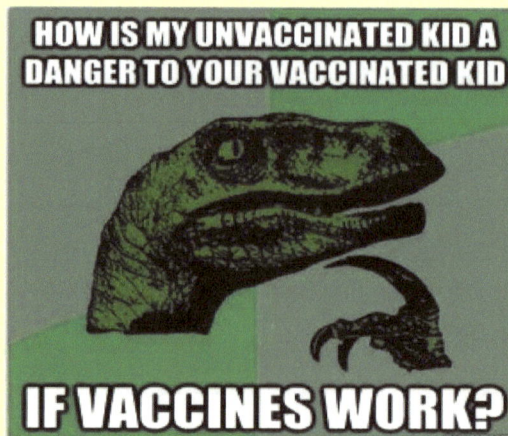

HOW IS MY UNVACCINATED KID A DANGER TO YOUR VACCINATED KID

IF VACCINES WORK?

This can be another motivation than profit health insurance is a continuous and large-scale criminal conspiracy, a policy of genocide against the population, representing, therefore, crimes against humanity that are internationally punishable by death.

 The fact that this goes before the wilfully international medical community makes it an international conspiracy in which the population has no recourse, given that vaccinations are becoming mandatory and are necessary conditions for many social programs.

 Persistent viruses and foreign proteins in the human body and their relationship to chronic and degenerative diseases was also raised by Dr. Robert Simpson of Rutgers University in 1976, when he addressed a seminar of researchers from the American Cancer Society, say "This pro-virus could be molecules in search of a disease."

Dr. Wendell Winters, a virologist at the University of California said "immunizations may cause changes in slow viruses and changes in the DNA mechanism."

Although host cells containing latent viral particles act more or less normally, they begin to synthesize viral proteins under the control of viral DNA, creating the circumstances for various autoimmune diseases, including diseases of the central nervous system, which, unfortunately, worse phenomenon increasing aberrant social behaviour.

World Health Organization has been criticized abroad for a number of experts, claiming that the WHO decision to declare pandemic was influenced by the pressures pharmaceutical companies eager to sell out to influenza vaccine.

Some of the vaccines side effects in Romania:

An increased incidence of children's cancer

The baby who was paralysed by a polio vaccine

Someone who was admitted to hospital in Cluj Napoca city of ROMANIA said that a whole floor was allocated to children with cancer. There are children with cancer starting three years old because of the vaccines! The Romanian hospital from Cluj-Napoca is full today with unhappy very young children with cancer.

Side effects of vaccines: flaccid

paraplegia (paralyse) after

vaccination

A baby in Slatina was paralysed

by a polio vaccine – (November

2011).

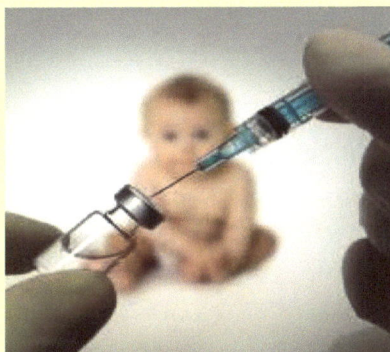

Just he was learning to walk, but he is paralysed from the waist down. We speak of a child of 14 months old. Disaster happened a day after the child has been vaccinated against polio. Doctors believe that baby has got very small chances of recovery and they sent him to Bucharest's doctors for further more tests.

The parents of the baby complain that the GP doctor has not done the vaccine properly. The vaccine was given by a nurse and supervised by a GP doctor in Schitu - River town. The parents of the baby said that after the vaccine has done, SUDDENLY, their child could not move the legs. The baby's parents were extremely desperate.

Their baby is crawling all day long from a bed to the other bed crying. " *I'd sell a kidney of mine just to see my child healthy again. After the vaccine was made, my frightened child is walking now like a snake...* " told to his neighbours very upset the father of the unhappy baby. The doctors called baby's illness as < **flaccid paraplegia>**, a disease that has dangerous consequences for all life.

The vaccination

has to reduce

the number of world population

The new "catastrophic" health, such as pandemic flu or swine flu, has been artificially created for humanity to be controlled more easily.

By creating panic among the population, through news alarming and worrisome statistics seeks to justify spending billions of dollars annually on the production of vaccines. Often, swine flu vaccination campaigns are introduced by force against the will of the population.

 But are these flu vaccines a saviour of life? This documentary film presents several cases in which **healthy people were incurably ill after being vaccinated. While the population dies or falls ill, the drug companies their profits get substantially thickens...**

You may see lots of information on the internet about "Bill and Melinda GATES FOUNDATIONS"" promoting poisonous vaccines all over the world to reduce the population of the planet...

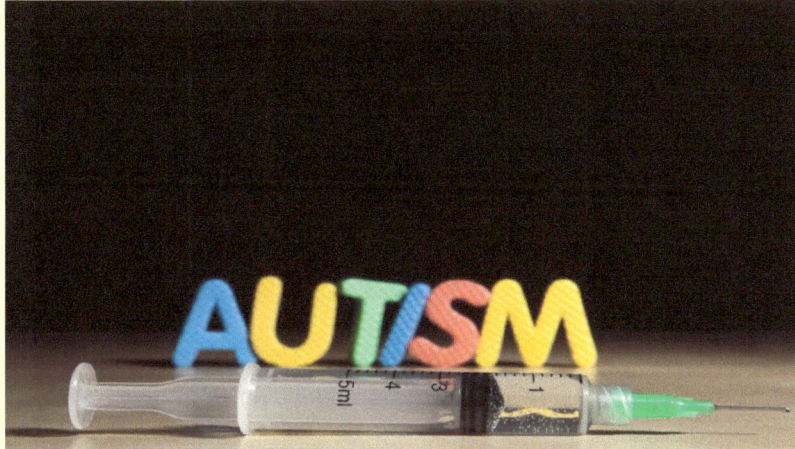

HERE IT IS ANOTHER PROOF : THIS MEDICAL STUDY

""As a physician, I found an explosion of diverse pathology in the young generation in spite of medical advances, progress in hygiene, food or comfort. Radioactivity in air, soil pollution, stress, diet can be drivers of different cancers in recent years.

But many emerging diseases in children are not due to pollution vaccine? More and more children complain of allergies, marked neurasthenia, flu, frequent colds, sleep disorders and gastrointestinal disorders.

Children may inherit some viruses but that is not evident in the elementary conditions of hygiene and nutrition, so no need to prevent disease through vaccination, but may acquire natural immunity to disease manifesting.

But if they are vaccinated, by disrupting the immune system can "awaken" these viruses "move", causing various diseases such as multiple sclerosis, cancer.

The practice of mandatory vaccination in 3rd world countries without taking into account the immune status of each individual (it is extremely dangerous, live or attenuated viruses are introduced into the body).

Smallpox: was eradicated following vaccination but not due to a higher standard of living (most cases were in Africa and Asia, and anyway epidemic was in decline when the vaccination campaign started).

At that time (1947 - 1979) vaccination caused more disease than smallpox itself. I. Teachers and B.Halibokowski Aleksandrowicz the Krakow Academy of Sciences published in "The Lancet" 1967: **"smallpox vaccination causes leukaemia".** Dr. B. Saint-Louis Hospital Duperre published in "La Presse Medical" in 1955: "smallpox vaccination causes leukaemia blast".

WHO program to eliminate the failed smallpox vaccination than after stopping.

For a period of 30 years many kids died from smallpox vaccination although there were also threatened by natural disease.

BCG (TB vaccine made at birth)

Dr. Scohy in "Des Clefs pour vivre" in August 1994 said: "It was found after vaccination worsening the pathological predispositions nose -pharyngitis, bronchitis, laryngitis and pave the way land and arthritic rheumatism."

After a study done in India in 1979, was reported by the WHO:

- BCG vaccination has no protective effect in the first 7.5 years after vaccination;

- BCG vaccination is already contested by 50 years, BCG vaccine inoculation is actually a very attenuated tuberculosis will grow up to 6-9 months. The next vaccine is usually two months that is in full tuberculosis.

For example a tetra- vaccine contains:

- Loffler bacillus toxins;

- Nicolair bacillus toxin;
- 5 billion of Bordetella pertussis bacilli in phase I ;
-> 100,000 polio virus type I inactivated with formalin;
-> 100,000 polio virus type II inactivated with formalin;
-> 300 000 Type III polio virus inactivated with formalin;

These doses are strictly the same, regardless of weight, age, state of immunity. Apply 3 kg infant as an adult of 80 kg without checking whether the patient can bear these poisons, viruses or bacilli.

The tetanus vaccine

Professor Tissot in 1947, said: "We know that a patient is never cured of tetanus immunized against a second infection and the serum is ineffective sold (can create a state of anaphylaxis even if a second infection) and produces and coli- bacillosis. Prevent tetanus is through proper cleaning and sanitizing infected wound.

DTTAB (vaccine against diphtheria, tetanus, typhoid). Statistically, it was found to cause nephritis, liver, and at 6 months after the vaccine may be found illness of typhoid fever. Produce sudden death in infants.

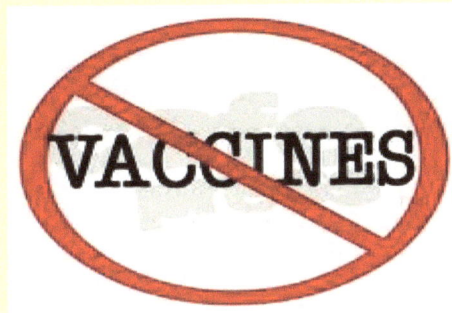

The Pertussis vaccine

Professor Rick from Middlesex hospital, leading authority in the field of immunology, said in 1973 in the Telegraph: **"multiple vaccines against pertussis and diphtheria can cause infirmity of many children, causing brain damage."** <u>Dr. Pilette</u> *Survive* in 1975 as quoted in "multiple vaccines against diphtheria, pertussis and polio may cause infirmity of the children".

Dr. Gordon T. Stewart Glasgow stating that 30% of cases of pertussis (WHOOPING COUGH) occur in vaccinated patients.

MMR vaccine (measles, mumps - rubella) were found in U.S. growth in 1990 despite constant high measles vaccination coverage. Official sources of mortality are 20 times higher than that of recorded before the introduction of the vaccine, pneumonia due to measles.

Slow viruses found in all vaccines and especially measles vaccine can hide human tissue and can occur later as complications: encephalitis, multiple sclerosis, ataxia, mental retardation, aseptic meningitis, diabetes, paralysis, Reye's syndrome. Squeal is the expression of encephalitis after vaccination attracting disruption of nerve maturation and attention deficit disorder, conduct disorder, autism.

According to W.H.O.: The chances of being contacted by the measles vaccinations are 15 times higher than in the non - vaccinated.

After MMR vaccinations there are side effects : arthritis, numbness in peripheral nerves may occur with delay up to 2 months after vaccination and that parents do not recognize the symptoms as being caused by the vaccine. Many parents of children in Great Britain refuse to vaccinate children with MMR as a new study has confirmed Crohm disease causing autism on those vaccinated. Dr. Helmke said that several months after vaccination against mumps can trigger diabetes.

The MMR vaccine strain URABE was withdrawn from the market on September 15, 1992 in Germany and the United Kingdom following the occurrence of cases of meningitis and Crohm disease. Despite this fact, in 2010 there were vaccines in London and Bromley surgeries ready to perform medical act to the children, GP and nurses ignores the danger of vaccinations. If childhood diseases occur naturally, it acquires a resistance of hereditary diseases such as asthma or eczema. In this respect, British and American researchers found that women who experienced natural mumps in childhood do not develop ovarian cancer in adulthood.

Hepatitis B vaccine produces immune disorders, hepatitis, meningitis, optic neuritis, seizures and epilepsy. In 1994 Pasteur - Mérieux had developed a hepatitis B vaccine taken in cultured hamster ovary cancer cells and thus to transmit individual vaccinated and cancer-virus (the virus responsible for cancer).

www. The British Medical Journal. co.uk **Live viruses introduced into the body as vaccine may recombine with viruses or defective retrovirus (not show) that already exist in the body and can generate a very dangerous hybrid virus. An expert made by INSERM (National Institute of Health - France) recognizes that vaccine efficacy ranging from 40-80%.**

In Switzerland, appeared 23 times more heads than facial nerve paralysis have been reported previously (Mutsch 2004). Polio vaccine - was taken from the monkey kidney tumour so vaccinated children contacted SV40 cancer virus which does not die in the chemical preservatives used to maintain the virus inside fluid immersion. Polio vaccine SABIN –was made from green monkey kidney (from Africa) contaminated with the virus STLV3 - forerunner of the origin of HIV AIDS.

WHO organization said that paralytic polio is the leading cause of disability in 3rd world countries and one in 10 dies from it. Of the polio vaccine is still given to children SABIN when Dr. Jonas Salk, who prepared the first polio vaccine in the world, shows that **the vaccine is one that causes most cases of polio illness.**

DTP vaccine (diphtheria-tetanus-pertussis) - is administered at 2, 4, 6, 12 months with a booster at 2 years and 6 months. Statistics after two thirds of deaths were sudden death in infants following DTP vaccination.

<u>**In U.S.A. children immunized against tetanus and chronic allergies contacted DTP two times longer than non- vaccinated children.**</u>

Interval	Vaccine	Effects
0-4 hours	All vaccines	Anaphylaxis, allergy
0-3 days	Whooping Cough	Encephalopathy, late - DZ
0-28 days	Tetanus	Plexus- brachialis-neuritis
5-15 days	ROR	Encephalitis
7-30 days	Rubella MMR	Thrombocytopenia
7-42 days	Rubella	Chronic arthritis,

<u>Today in Germany there is NO compulsory vaccination for childre</u>, as has been reported after vaccination 1995-2004 annual severe disability (60% were **compensated).**

All international statistics show various falsifications because vaccinations have been sustained interest and ignorance of the events after vaccination.

They spend more money for vaccine propaganda than their long-term research. To deceive public opinion and health professionals, vaccine manufacturers show descending curve after introduction of the vaccine, but really strong infectious disease was declining before vaccination and their introduction caused outbreaks of disease that must be immunized against.

<u>Please to reflect on the increasing number of cases of cancer and diabetes.</u>

 The principle of mandatory vaccinations would have never accepted the government because it is contrary to basic human rights. It is the failure of opinion and individual liberties.""

(source : MD, Mihailescu, Gavriil, ATITUDINI Magazine, no.10, 2010 , Romanian public domain).

REFERENCES :

   ☐☐   Kaufmann (RE) and Janeway (M.), quoted in the article by Pilette, La poliomyélite [Poliomyelitis - bluntly], in Survive, 1975, page 26;

   ☐☐   Montanari (G.): male di Stato epilettico susseguente the first is seconded iniezione Salk polio con vaccino typo [status epilepticus successive first and second injections Salk polio vaccine type - bluntly], in "Minerva Medica ", no. 54/ August 1962; Baguley (DM) and Glasgow (GL): Subacute sclerosing Panencephalitis and the Salk Vaccine [subacute sclerosing panencephalitis and Salk vaccine - bluntly], in "The Lancet", October 6, 1973;

   ☐☐   Hinton (GG) et coll.: After Oral Poliomyelitis Vaccine paralysis [Paralysis after Oral polio vaccine - bluntly], in the Canadian Medical Association Journal [-n.tr. Canadian Medical Association Journal], no. 87 October 1962;

   ☐☐   Bojitiov (S.) et coll.: Encéphalo-myélo-suite de l'polyradiculonévrites and utilisation antipoliomyclitique Sabin vaccine avec germ vivant [Encefalo-myelo-poliradiculonevritele as a result of using Sabin polio vaccine with seed alive - bluntly] , in "La Presse Medical

[Medical Press - bluntly]", no. 72, January 11, 1964;

☐☐ Orstavik (I.) et coll.: Paralytic Poliomyelitis in Norway Since the Introduction of the Trivalent Oral Vaccine [Paralytic poliomyelitis in Norway since the introduction of trivalent oral vaccine - bluntly], in Bull.OMS, 1971;

☐☐ Aaby, P., Jensen, H., Gomes, J., Fernandes, M., Lisse, IM: The Introduction of diphtheria tetanus-pertussis vaccine and Child Mortality in Rural Guinea-Bissau: an observational study. Int J Epidimiol 2004, 33 (2): 374-380;

☐☐ Aaby, P., Vessari, H., Nielsen, J., Kenneth, M., et al: Sex differential effects of routine immunizations and childhood survival in rural Malawi. Ped Infect Dis J 2006, 25 (8): 721-727;

☐☐ *August.* Albonico, H., et al.: Febrile infectious childhood diseases in the history of cancer Patients and matched controls. Med Hypotheses, 1998c, 51 (4): 315-320;

☐☐ *September.* Bach, JF: The Effect of Infections on Susceptibility to autoimmune and allergic Disease (Review). N Engl J Med 2002, 347: 911-920;

☐☐☐ Barlow, WE, Davis RL, Glasser, JW, Rhodes, PH: The risk of seizures after receipt of whole-cell pertussis or measles, mumps, and rubella vaccine V. N Engl J Med 2001, 345 (9): 656-661 Barr, R., Limp, K.: Measles Fact Sheet. Autism independent United Kingdom, 1999.

☐☐☐ Bergfors, E., Bjorkelund, C, Trollfors, B.: Nineteen Cases of persistent prudential ritic nodules and contact allergy to aluminum after injection of aluminum-adsorbed Commonly Used Vaccines. Eur J Pediatr 2005, 164 (11): 691-7;

☐☐☐ Bernsen, RM: Childhood asthma and allergy: the role of vaccinations and Other Early life events.EUR, Medical, Dissertations, 2005. http://repub eur.nl/publications/med_hea/mh3/229957523 /

☐☐☐ Böhlke, K., Davis RL, Marcy, SM, Braun, MM, et al.: Risk of anaphylaxis after vaccination of children and adolescents. Pediatrics 2003, 112 (4): 815-820;

☐☐☐ Burmistrova, AL Gorshunova, LP, Ebert, L.: Change in the non-specific resistance of the body, or to influenza and acute respiratory diseases diphtheria-tetanus vaccines Following immunization diphtheria-tetanus vaccine. Zh Mikrobiol Immunobiol Epidemiol 1976 (3): 89-91;

☐☐☐ CDC (Centers for Disease Control and Prevention): thiomersal in Vaccines: a joint statement of the American Academy of Pediatrics and the Public Health Service r. MMWR 1999, 48 (26): 563-565;

☐☐☐ Centers for Disease Control and Prevention): Overview of vaccine safety. In 2003. http://www.cdc.gov/nip/vacsafe/

☐☐☐ Cizman, M., et al.: Aseptic meningitis after measles vaccination Against * and mumps. Pediatric Infectious Disease Journal 1989, 8: 302-308;

☐☐☐ DuVernoy, TS, Braun, MM: Hypotonic-hyporesponsive episodes Reported to the Vaccine

Adverse Event Reporting System (VAERS), 1996-1998. Pediatrics 2000, 106 (4): E52;

☐☐☐ EURODIAB ACE Study Group: Variation and trends in child-hood Incidence of diabetes in Europe. Lancet 2000, 355: 873-876;

☐☐☐ Farwell JR, Dohrmann, GJ, Marrett, LD, Meigs, JW: Effect of SV40 virus-contaminated polio vaccine on the Incidence and type of CNS neoplasms in children: a Population-based study. Trans Am Neurol I-shock, 1979, 104: 261-264;

☐☐☐ Fisher MA, Eklund SA, James SA, Lin, X.: Adverse Events Associated with Hepatitis B vaccine in U.S. children Less than six years of age, 1993 and 1994. Ann Epidemiol 2001, 11 (1): 13-21;

☐☐☐ Griffin MR, et al.: Risk of seizures and encephalopathy after immunization with Diphtheria-Tetanus-Pertussis the vaccine. I Med J 1990 Association, 263: 1641-1645;

☐☐☐ Harrison, BJ, Thomson, W., Pepper, L., Ollier, WE: Patients who Develop * inflammatory polyarthritis (IP) after immunization is clinically indistinguishable from Other Patients with IP. Br J Rheumatol 1997, 36 (3) :366-369;

☐☐☐ Hernan, MA, Jick, SS, Olek, MJ, Jick, H: Recombinant Hepatitis B vaccine and the risk of multiple sclerosis: A prospective study. Neurology 2004, 63:723-772;

☐☐☐ HORNIG, M., Chian, D., Lipkin, WI: neurotoxic effects of thiomersal has postnatal mouse strain dependent. Molecule Psychiatry 2004: 1-13;

☐☐☐ Jefferson T, Rudin, M., Di Pietrantoni, C.: Adverse events after aluminum-containing DTP immunisation with Vaccines: Systematic Review of the Evidence. Lancet Infect Dis 2004, 4 (2): 84-90;

☐☐☐ Lee, R., Robinson JL, Spady, DW: Frequency of apnea, bradycardia, and desaturations following and diphtheria-tetanus-pertussis first-inactivated polio-Haemophilus influenzae type B immunization in hospitalized Infants. BMC Pediatr 2006: 6: 20;

☐☐☐ Miller, E., Andrews, N., Stowe, J., Grant, A., et al: Risk of aseptic meningitis convulsed and measles-mumps-rubella Following vaccination in the United Kingdom. Am J Epidemiol 2007, 165 (6): 704-709;

☐☐☐ Montgomery, SM, Morris DL, Pounder RE, et al.: Paramyxoviruses Infections in childhood inflammatory bowel disease and Subsequent. Gastroenterology 1999, 116 (4): 796-803;

☐☐☐ Petrik, MS, Wong, M. C, Tabata, R. C, Garry, RF, Shaw, CA: Aluminium adjuvant linked to Gulf War Illness induces motor neuron death in mice. Neuromoleeular Med 2007, 9 (1): 83-100;

☐☐☐ Valerian, V: Developmental neurobiology contraindicates vaccine paradigm. The mechanism of encephalitic damage from Vaccines. 2000, http :/ / www. trafax. org / vaccines / myelin.html;

☐☐☐ Verstraeten T, Davis RL, DeStefano, F., Lieu, TA, et al.: Safety of thiomersal-containing Vaccines: a two-phased study of computerize health maintenance Organization databases. Pediatrics 2003, 112 (5): 1039-1048;

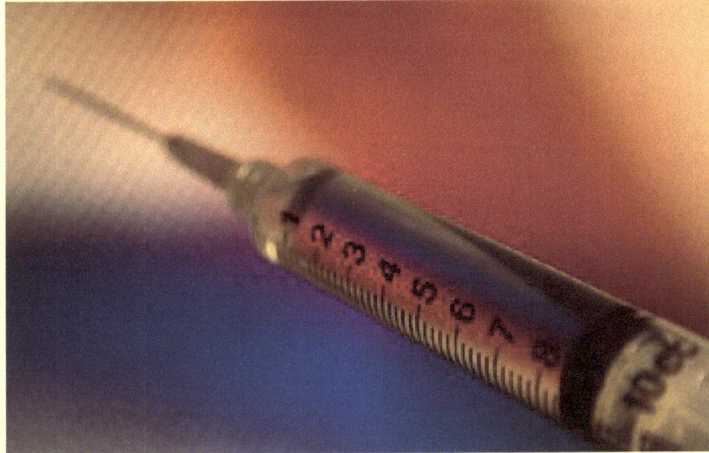

Why You Should Never
Vaccinate Infants and Children

"There is no scientific studies to determine whether vaccines have really prevented diseases. Rather disease graphs show vaccines have been introduced at the fag end of epidemics when the disease was already in its last stages. In case of Small Pox the vaccine actually caused a great spurt in the incidence of disease killing thousands before public outcry led to its withdrawal.

There are no long-term studies on vaccine safety. Very short-term unscientific tests are carried out where the vaccinated subjects are checked against another group who are given another vaccine.

Technically the tests should be carried out against a non-vaccinated group. No one really knows what protocols are followed at such industry-sponsored trials.

There has never been any attempt to compare a vaccinated population against a non vaccinated population to know what vaccines are doing to the children and the society.

The child receives not one but many vaccines. There are no tests to determine the effects of multiple vaccines.

There is no scientific basis for vaccinating infants. As per senior doctors quoted by the Times of India, "Children suffer from less that 2% of vaccine preventable illnesses but 100% of the vaccines are targeted towards them." The vaccine pioneers who have recommended abundant caution before vaccinating the population have never advocated Mass vaccinations.

Vaccinating infants is the most profitable business both for the manufacturers as well as the doctors.

ALL THE VACCINE INGREDIENTS ARE EXTREMELY TOXIC IN NATURE.

Vaccines contain heavy metals, cancer causing substances, toxic chemicals, live and genetically modified viruses, contaminated serum containing animal viruses and foreign genetic material, extremely toxic decontaminates and adjutants, untested antibiotics, none of which can be injected without causing any harm.

The mercury, aluminum and live viruses in vaccines is behind the huge epidemic of autism (1 in 10 worldwide as per doctors in the USA), a fact that has been admitted by the US Vaccine Court.

The CDC of USA, the vaccine watchdog, has publicly admitted that its much-publicized 2003 study denying any link between vaccines and autism, is flawed. The Chief of CDC Dr Gerberding has confessed to the media (CNN) that vaccines can cause "autism like symptoms". The Autism epidemic is found only in those countries that have allowed mass vaccinations.

In the year 1999, the US Government instructed vaccine manufacturers to remove mercury from vaccines "with immediate effect". But mercury still remains a part of many vaccines. The vaccines with mercury were never recalled and were given to children up to the year 2006. "Mercury free" vaccines contain 0.05mcg of mercury, enough to permanently damage a infant.

Mercury used in vaccines is second in toxicity only to the radioactive substance, Uranium. It is a neurologically - toxin that can damage the entire nervous system of the infant in no time.

Mercury accumulates in fat. The brain being made entirely of fat cells, most of the mercury accumulates there giving rise to the peculiar symptoms of the autistic children.

The mercury used in vaccines is ethyl mercury. According to Indian doctors this is 1000 times more toxic than the usual methyl mercury.

The aluminum present in vaccines makes the mercury, in any form, 100 times more toxic.

As per an independent study aluminum and formaldehyde present in vaccines can increase the toxicity of mercury, in any form, by 1000 times.

A child is receiving 250 times more mercury through vaccines than they can possibly tolerate. The same article states that if one considers the WHO limit for mercury in water, they are receiving 50,000 times the limit. The limits set, incidentally, are for adults and not infants.

Autism in India has emerged as the most rapidly growing epidemic amongst children. From 1 in 500 it has steadily climbed to 1 in 37 today. As per Indian doctors, "You can go to any class of any school today and find an autistic child."

Autism is a permanent disability that affects the child physically, mentally and emotionally. It makes the child loose social contact. It impedes both the physical and mental growth of the child. It destroys the brain causing severe memory and attention problems.

According to vaccine researcher Dr Harris Coulter, vaccines cause children to become pervert and criminal. All the school shootings by the children in the USA are by autistic children. Vaccines can cause more harm that even the medical community privately acknowledges.

Autistic children also suffer from severe bowel disorders. As per Dr Andrew Wakefield, this is due to the vaccine strain live measles virus in the MMR vaccine. Nearly all children become fully autistic after the MMR shot.

The DPT also causes children to regress giving rise to fears that multiple live virus vaccines are an important cause behind autism. If three live viruses can cause so much harm we can well imagine what today's five and seven viruses vaccines will do to children.

Before the autism epidemic, it is already well known that vaccines have caused the cancer epidemic in today's society. Both the Small Pox and the Oral Polio Vaccine are made from monkey serum. This serum has helped many cancer causing monkey viruses, 60 found so far, to enter the human blood stream.

It is also known that it is the use of green monkey serum in vaccines that has led to the transfer of the Sivian Immune deficiency Virus (SIV) from monkeys into humans. The SIV and the HIV that causes AIDS are very similar.

Not only AIDS, a blood cancer in infants (Acute Lymphoblastic Leukemia) that is affecting children in thousands is also due to the extremely toxic nature of vaccine ingredients.

Infantile jaundice and also infantile diabetes is also scientifically connected to the toxic vaccines.

The live polio viruses used in the Oral Polio Vaccine has caused Vaccine Attributed Paralytic Polio in more than 65,000 children as per doctors of the Indian Medical Association. In the USA this vaccine has caused polio 16 years after administration. The OPV has also let loose a new strain of polio in both India and Africa. The OPV is banned in other countries.

Vaccines contain serum from not only chimpanzees and monkeys but also from cows, pigs, chickens, eggs, horses, and even human serum and tissues extracted from aborted fetuses.

Deaths and permanent disability from vaccines is very common and known by the medical community. They are instructed by the Government to keep quiet and not to associate such cases with vaccines.

Many doctors argue that diseases during childhood are due to the body exercising its immune system. Suppressing these diseases causes the immune system to remain undeveloped causing the various autoimmune disorders like diabetes and arthritis that have become epidemics today.

Vaccines suppress the natural immunity and the body does not have natural antibodies anymore. The mothers milk therefore does not contain natural antibodies and can no longer protect the child against illnesses.

In the USA vaccine adverse effects are recorded and the Government offers compensation of millions of dollars to victims (the most recent case in its Vaccine Court may have received up to $200 million in damages). The Indian Government simply refuses to acknowledge that vaccines can cause deaths and permanent disability.

It has been scientifically proven that vaccines cannot prevent disease. We still do not know enough about the human immune system and therefore we should not interfere with it.

The BCG vaccine for tuberculosis has been extensively tested in India as long back as 1961 and found to be totally ineffective.

The OPV is causing polio and other neurological and intestinal disorders in tens of thousands of Indian children. The Hep-B vaccine introduced recently is not meant for children at all, it is a vaccine for a sexually transmitted disease that should be targeted only at promiscuous adults.

The doctors themselves avoid the DPT as it is one of the most toxic vaccines ever devised. The measles vaccine is a vaccine that regularly causes severe adverse effects and the health workers want it out.

The Rotavirus vaccine, Hib vaccine, HPV vaccine and the various multiple various vaccines being introduced without any kind of testing is only because the vaccine manufacturers and the doctors administering them want to ensure a good income.

 If after reading all this information you still want to vaccinate your child, please go ahead. You deserve a vaccine-damaged child! "" (SOURCE: Jagannath Chatterjee.).

DECLARATION OF A DOCTOR

"It is now 30 years since I have been confining myself to the treatment of chronic diseases. During those 30 years I have run against so many histories of little children who had never seen a sick day until they were vaccinated and who, in the several years that have followed, have never seen a well day since. I couldn't put my finger on the disease they have. They just weren't strong.   Their resistance was gone. They were perfectly well before they were vaccinated.
They have never been well since. "---

Dr. William Howard Hay

THE INTERNATIONAL DEVIL ORGANIZATION -

"W.H.O." IS VERY SMART INDEED

TO KILL CHILDREN!

The "let's destroy people's health" organization W.H.O. recommends vaccines to "**people with risks**" like the following ones:

- **people aged over 65 years;**

- **people (children, youth, adults & seniors) with chronic medical conditions (lung and heart),**

- **people (children, youth, adults and seniors) with chronic metabolic diseases (diabetes, renal dysfunction, haemoglobin disorders, immune- suppression);**

- **medical staff;**

- **workers in essential community services: customs officers, fire-fighters, police, military etc., students and other people living in dormitories**

- **families of those affected;**

- **The second and third trimester pregnant women in pregnancy. (It is very dangerous to make vaccines on pregnant women!!!)**

IF YOU NOTICED THEY ARE TARGETING ALL PEOPLE FROM SOCIETY!

If the failed Tamiflu (a drug used in influenza, because of which many people died), is trying to influenza vaccine. But "if a true pandemic, not to have any chance," says Johannes van der Wouden, expert in epidemiology flu (influenza) from Erasmus University in Rotterdam.

He refers to the fact that currently uses the same mode of preparation of influenza vaccine in the past: the influenza virus is propagated in living embryo, chicken. But really aggressive virus would immediately destroy the living organisms and small. "If the virus would be so aggressive and would kill them, it is possible for people not to get employees to work the next day ..." he says. (**source :Ehgartner, Bert., Lob der Krankheit, 2004, page 277).**

Van der Wouden critical and how the WHO (World Health Organization) control and monitor the development and prevention of influenza (Influenza) using the 112 regulations in 83 countries!

The studies show there but something else…

Tom Jefferson, coordinator of the group, summarizes, writing that ***"for children under two years vaccines have placebo effect (none), and for elderly people is better to wash their hands more often and have a style healthy life than to go to the doctor to get vaccinated.***
"(Jefferson says the girl where is the problem:" It is time for those who are in WHO's Lobby and the Ministry of Health of the U.S. to be removed because experts from the flu (influenza) people recommend their products - like they do and those who sell vacuum cleaners to get rid of merchandise - as if we all a mob of *idiots. "(ibid., 278).* Jefferson wants to emphasize through this last statement he makes, and lack of quality education, especially in people over 65 years, studies that used them to his analysis.

The results show two things that contradict: *on the one hand to the vaccinated protection from flu is virtually zero (!) And on the other hand, vaccination would decrease the risk of death. But that would mean that the vaccine actually appears to the elderly other diseases such as diabetes, stroke, etc., but not the flu, which is nonsense! (Tom Jefferson, Carlo D.- "Inactivated Influenza Vaccines in the elderly - are you sure?", Lancet 2007, 370:1199-1200).*

Studies, said Jefferson, are made in a totally disproportionate: the vaccine are mostly healthy people and control group (those UN-vaccinated) is represented in most cases of flu that old sick feeling very weak and sick to go to the doctor. So, no wonder that there are many deaths in this group of people.

 Flu deaths are fortunately very rare in children. In Germany statistics show that children under five years, was one death in 2005 and in 2004 were 2 cases. **But this is not due to vaccines. We find in this age group a total influenza vaccine ineffective.** For this reason, Jefferson and colleagues have written to all 30 study groups and have asked any secondary reactions of the vaccine in children. Some scientists have said that indeed there are such studies, but the company producing the vaccine did not want to make public any such study. **"Hence there is a danger that some rare side reactions of the vaccine is not yet well studied"** Jefferson critical attitude vaccine manufacturers. (source : *Jefferson T et al. "Safety of Influenza Vaccines in Children", Lancet 2005, 366: 803-804).*

Influenza vaccination for the **pregnant women** could not ever give immunity to the child . (France 2006).

Side effects of influenza vaccine are :

- *Local and general symptoms:*

- local pain;

- flu-like symptoms: muscle and joint pain, tiredness (fatigue), headache, fever (Thurairajan 1997);

- These symptoms affect a rate of 14% in children aged between 11 and 15 years (Neuzil 2002); *symptoms increase gradually with age and also lower immunity to other respiratory infections and other diseases,* child consultations to family physicians multiply long after the flu shot (Hoberman 2003).

Allergic reactions and circulatory disorders

- vaccine can cause *mild allergic reactions to allergic shock,* especially to hen egg proteins that vaccine virus is grown, they are among allergic people to the egg but they can also induce such an allergy for the first time; (Yamani 1998) ;

- *syndrome "respiratory"* is another form of allergy vaccine is the emergence of a form of conjunctivitis, facial oedema and respiratory distress;

Asthma

- Although there is no proven beneficial effect of influenza vaccine in patients with asthma, they are the group "at risk" in which influenza vaccination is recommended after STIKO and the other health institutions in the world. Is it so? *In adults* was observed in one study to those vaccinated worsening asthma (Cates 1999) and *in children,* studies show that after vaccination increased frequency of asthma: two studies done in 1300 shows an increase in children vaccinated frequency of asthma and in one study even a doubling of the disease group compared with non-vaccinated children (Bueving 2004, Christy 2004);

- *allergic asthma cases occur after several years of vaccination* (Takahashi 2007).

Autoimmune diseases

- was observed that after vaccination is sometimes an autoimmune reaction by forming antibodies against its own cells (Stepanova 2000);

- medical literature we find many cases of autoimmune disease affecting blood vessels and kidneys *(vasculitis),* attributed to influenza vaccine components (Yanai-Berar 2002, Tavadia 2003); *adjutant MF 59* apparently can induce a *lupus erythematosus* (Satos 2003), and various nerve complications are due to the flu shot.

Neurological complications

- *Thiomersalului present in the vaccine as a preservative* (thiomersal contains mercury, organic nerve shown in percentage of 49, 6%!) is *a real nervous system toxicity* and which, being gathered every year in those vaccinated (especially the elderly and children) can lead to serious diseases, nerve;

- The flu vaccine can cause people with a genetic predisposition to an autoimmune reaction against brain tissue, leading to de-myelination it, therefore there is a more or less damage important

50

nerves or neurons (nerve cells) or spinal cord; a serious *acute demyelinating encephalomyelitis* represents (Nakamura 2003);

- *infections* were described *nerve* pain and functional disorders, especially of the hands or face (Felix 1976, Schumm 1976, Ehrengut 1977, Furlow 1977, Hennessen 1978). The optic nerve *disorders appear to* the eye muscle paralysis, double vision or strabismus (Hennessen 1977, Kawasaki 1998);

- *Guillain-Barre syndrome* is a serious side effect, the dreaded influenza vaccine. Link between the disease and vaccine has been proven and recognized (Bryan 1977, Juurlink 2006, Souayah 2007). Between 1991-1999, the U.S. 382 cases were reported, most of cases beginning in the3 first 2 weeks of vaccination in 2004 were announced 31 cases which started in the first 6 weeks of the shot (Souayah 2007). Frequency of this syndrome is 4 times higher than after DTP after flu vaccine (Geier 2003); It has been reported other nervous disorders such as *bladder dysfunction, disturbances in sexual dynamics, dizziness and gait disturbance (Wells* 1971, Ehrengut 1977, Hennessen 1977, Poser 1982, Bakshi 1996).

The H1N1 flu vaccine Pandemrix commissioned by the Ministry of Health to immunize children was refused several European countries because it has side effects. Swedish media reported that six patients have died of swine flu because vaccination with Pandemrix.

In addition, Pandemrix has caused disputes in Sweden after 350 people were immunized with this drug have experienced side effects. But conspiracy of vaccines reached its peak in Finland, where the former Minister of Health accuses world leaders to use H1N1 vaccine to decrease the population. "It is dangerous H1N1 type flu but vaccine. It is very toxic and made to bring billions and billions into the pockets of those who manufacture vaccine, "said the former Minister of Health, DR. Rauni Kilda. http://www.youtube.com/watch?feature=player_embedded&v=185HKE2c5Gg

Does Vaccination makes sense?

About side effects of compounds in vaccines

We are speaking about the 5th Symposium on vaccines from July 16, 2009 - Stuttgart / in Germany

a) "Side effects of the compounds of the vaccine"

DR. Klaus Hartmann spent 10 years at the Paul-Ehrlich Institute in Germany. At many conferences where he was invited, tell us about his experience in the field of vaccines, especially focusing on the components side effects of vaccines.

Main ideas of the conference about these side effects:

The mercury (from various sources such as *amalgam of fillings, thiomersal,* etc.) on nervous system development was studied first by a University of Medicine in Calgary - California, the study being funded only by faculty, and thus a private study without the contribution of institutions of interest as pharmaceutical companies, chemical industry, etc..). (See YouTube video study: http://embedr.com/playlist/5-6-stuttgarter-impfsymposium).

This study was published in 2001 in local Medical Journal has aroused the interest of many scientists. The study shows how normal the first year of life the child develops new neurons (nerve cells and their extensions) and neuronal synapses (connections between neurons), by stimulating nerve cells that process <u>itself.</u> <u>When you pour mercury (much less than that contained in the vaccines!), We see how these connections not forward but rather break, is a definitive trial!</u>

Therefore do not develop a large number of nerve connections that can not only have a disastrous effect on nervous system development in children. Unfortunately we have no studies showing nerve development long after.

<u>It was noted that Thiomersal decomposes into its components (mercury + GTP) in the human brain,</u> where mercury is released, it works the same way described above on nerve cells.

For the vaccine to take effect proposed, is needed to induce an "infection" of the virus in the vaccine. If the virus used is "alive" will be so-called "original infection" and if the virus is dead or is it of toxins (for example the tetanus) requires a third component "dirty secret" called <u>adjutant</u> which infection induces an "artificial".

The tetanus vaccine adjutant is a compound of <u>aluminium (aluminium hydroxide) which is considered a necessary adjunct, without which there is no immunological reaction!</u> (?!)

Note: *DR. Klaus Hartmann <u>Aluminium</u> assign the role of <u>"adjutant"</u> for vaccine without immune stimulation does not occur, unlike those who promote vaccines and which he considers to be preserved even rule out that it would have toxic effects on the nervous system.*

Regardless of the vaccine virus (live or attenuated / dead), will be induced infection in the body and other substances in the vaccine (aluminium) will destroy neurons and their connections.

So you made such as ["Gulf War Syndrome"](), when it was found actually surprised that this syndrome suffered not only soldiers leave Iraq, but soldiers who were trained in America but not the war had gone! In all of whom they were made more specific vaccines to prevent infections in the Gulf, including tetanus. All vaccines contained aluminium. Largest aluminium content in the vaccine had "anthrax" given to the soldiers.

It is known that a vaccine without preservatives and additives have no major effect on the immune system! Therefore these substances need to create a state of immunity from infection. The dormant-attenuated viruses from vaccines cannot survive without mercury or AL(OH)3.

b) "Safety of vaccines?"

Dr. med. Klaus Hartmann speaks from experience living in the Paul Ehrlich Institute (IPE) in Germany about how "safe" are vaccinations.

The doctor tells us that whenever they happen to be challenged by serious side effects of vaccines, the explanation is always the *same:* *"It is pure coincidence, there is no vaccine now!"* It is all a coincidence that the health management organization known EMEA (European Medicines Agency) is none other than Mr. Gunter Verheugen's?

One). We know about this man that has nothing to do with the medical and vaccine research, but has a high function, *European Commissioner for Enterprise* and *Industry and Vice President of* the *European Commission,* making the connection between vaccines and Chemical Industry Mafia! EMEA is to "make law" for the European Union, it depends if a vaccine is approved or not. It should be noted that "one of the Paul-Ehrlich Institute cannot oppose the use of a vaccine" Any request made to the EMEA is always rejected! EMEA is to prepare the "fertile ground" for the vaccine manufacturer. This is the only mechanism that works by EMEA.

Often those employed in IPE we wonder that a vaccine or drug to a wide range of dangerous side effects could be put on the market, but this always happens without anyone still angry or comment. Recently an article appeared about "safe vaccines" in Germany, written by a member of the Paul-Ehrlich Institute and Dr. Burkhard Schneeweiss (working at *Glaxo-Smith-Kline Company*!) Who write only about the safety of vaccines, without give any other explanation (recognition of side effects, their sorting, searching and removing their causes, etc.) using the lack of knowledge and experience of those from other areas?

Two.) Dr.med. Georg : "What should I do for my children's health?" *This doctor has an office in Munich where his wife, using natural treatments, treating patients who became ill because of vaccines. Patients presenting to their office in Germany and other European countries, which suffer from serious diseases caused by vaccines but could not be cured with medicines . He describes some of the serious cases children treated but he initiated the practice and prevention programs for these diseases.*

Neuro- dermitis is one of serious diseases caused by vaccines. It is very severe skin lesions in children (see picture on youtube). I noticed that this injury occurs especially after _Hexavaccinul_ given to children. One of the first cases that came to me in my office was a boy of 3-4 years whose disease started at age 2-3 months. Her face was full of wounds but was also very nervous, because suffering and ADHD *((attention deficit / hyperkinetic disorder)* were 3 adults need to be kept under control. Many serious cases were also presented to me in my office that had failed all medical treatment in different medical institutions in the country and abroad. I started in all these children a natural treatment.

Psoriasis is another consequence of vaccines. We observed very large and very severe forms in children. It is known that this disease is chronic and there is no effective conventional treatment.

Uncontrollable muscle contractions (similar to the tetanus), is another serious condition that occurs after Hexa- vaccine. A girl in Vienna contractions occurred after the second dose at age 6 months Hexa- vaccine. He <u>is 50 contractions</u> p <u>/ day,</u> severe mental retardation and motor, could not communicate at all with it. After treatment for these contractions disappeared and the girl who is now 8 or 9 years can go sit in the ass and even supported but there is no chance of communication with her.

Three.) Friedrich Klammrodt: teacher

"ADHD *(attention deficit / hyper kinetic disorder)* - side effects of vaccines?"

This teacher is a father of three children suffering from this syndrome and, in an attempt to treat children, noted a link between vaccines and these diseases. He is the organizer of the symposium in Stuttgart.

This syndrome was not known in the past when there were still no vaccine and in the years 1972-76 when there were a total of only 5 vaccines in total, combined between them. This syndrome has emerged after the introduction of a number of mandatory vaccines (especially combined) in infants and children. See the brief history of vaccines:

- Further increased the number of vaccines to _14, then 32!_

_- In 1995_ is _used trivaccinul (3 vaccines combined),_ then _tetravaccinul (4 vaccines combined!)._

- In 2006 it was 40 one child vaccine doses were administered between 1-6 years! In 2006 it introduced _for the first time hexavaccinul infant (6 vaccines at once!). For this year, the frequency of ADHD greatly increases ._

4.) Hans Tolzin - German journalist "Swine flu and pandemic artificial"

This time I want to make _a parallel between the 3 flu "pandemic" current swine flu, swine flu and the 1976 Spanish flu of 1917._ All three have a common flu: initially appeared to soldiers, so young and healthy men , to the surprise of scientists, then was extended to the general population. Flu "swine" would be defined today as "Mexican flu", the place where he "appeared" so called "pandemic". This flu was already known since 1976 when, due to a single death of a soldier (who died probably due to saturation than influenza) were vaccinated 40 million soldiers! _Mrs. Bean_ who _Eleanore I.Mc_ was there, tells us in her many writings that 500 soldiers were paralysed and 30 died from swine flu vaccines. All these soldiers were vaccinated with the flu shortly before important!

We know that there are special laboratories of the Army they are "grown" such viruses "pandemic".

Organization WHO (World Health Organization) is involved in "creating" current "swine flu pandemic artificial". WHO is an organization subordinate to the CDC (Center for Disease Control in the U.S.). _CDC may declare a state whenever and wherever a pandemic!_

5.) Dr. Jenö Ebert: "A controversial Nobel Prize!"

Ebert is a physician and internist . Dr.Jenö reveals some interesting facts about the Nobel Prize granted German doctor Harald zur Hausen (for discovery HPV) and about possible corruption related to awarding this prize.

Astra-Zeneca Company has a contract with people who give Nobel prizes. This company is actually the main sponsor for Nobel prizes. The company earned 200 million euros in 2007 in business for infection with HPV vaccine! How? Bo Angelin is the management company and Astra-Zeneca is also member of the Nobel Prize and B.Friedholm - Chairman of the Committee - the two largest contracts filed by Astra-Zeneca in 2006. Commission Secretary - Prof. Hans-Jörwall, was the only one admitted that it had "serious doubts" regarding the "legality" of the award given to the discovery of HPV, saying it could be an economic interest ...

Of those who realized the existence of corruption, was also Mrs. Christa van der Knast - Attorney General Anti-corruption Department of State in Sweden - which filed a complaint concerning possible corruption linked to the Nobel Prize given to Prof. Harald zur Hausen. The news appeared on October 12.). 2008 and TAZ (www.taz.de).

Dr. Jenö Ebert tells us about the secondary reactions of vaccines directed against HPV?

A U.S. study conducted by VAERS (Vaccine Adverse Event Reporting System) about vaccine side effects created against HPV shows that between July 2006 - April 2009, on a sample of 13,422 children vaccinated against HPV, in 15% of cases were serious side reactions such as: severe disorders of vision, paralysis and Guillain- Barré syndrome. The statistics show that autoimmune diseases occur three times more common (compared to the NON - vaccinated), and from 42 pregnant women inadvertently vaccinated (!) aborted 18! All This study shows that there were VAERS deaths were due to the vaccine: 22 deaths in 2007, 16 in 2008 and 3 in 2009! Many deaths have occurred because of other vaccines!

5.) Bert Ehgartner - Austrian journalist: "Tick hunt people ..."

Deliberately created a state of panic related to a human infection caused by tick. It's _borreliosis, or Lyme's disease called Lyme recurrent fever._ Due to excessive publicity, seems out of Hitchcock's

films, people feel "threatened" the poor animals called tick which overnight became "a monster". People are afraid to step on a field in May or to walk with their children in parks for fear of meeting with this monster. Only purpose of this theater is the vaccine? Vaccine was produced for the first time in Austria by Dr. Kunz . But soon they began to side effects of this vaccine. When the Austrian company, which then monopolize the market with a single existing vaccine against infection on tick, the company was acquired by Baxter who created a subsidiary in Heidelberg in Germany. Thus the vaccine has spread to Germany. Unfortunately, vaccine side effects are not recognized by any STIKO (Commission for vaccines) in Germany.

We all know that, _whatever the methods used, the flu contagiousness can never be controlled_ by any vaccine, especially in today's conditions when travel the world in hours from end to end.

But it is not _a normal state_ when the event of an outbreak of flu, ill only 5-10% of the population, and a rate of 90-95% remain healthy? This shows that in fact it creates a natural immunity to infection, and any epidemic is declining at a time and disappears. This is normal and natural.

Source: http://embedr.com/playlist/5-6-stuttgarter-impfsymposium

If vaccines have eradicated epidemic,

why are people now manages outbreaks?

Therefore believe that the government closes our increasingly more contracts for millions and millions of Euro with Big Pharma (big pharmaceutical companies) in our health care, to keep us from epidemics of diphtheria, tetanus, whooping cough (pertussis), mumps, rubella and measles to TB, of polio, hepatitis, etc.. ?

Let's face it! The first three listed diseases are treated with ...

ordinary penicillin (Amoxicillin, Augmentin, etc..), Mumps, rubella and measles patiently terrible ravages TB (7000 deaths per year) even though we Ultra vaccinated with BCG, polio has disappeared, and hepatitis is transmitted only through blood and other fluids every case is preventable by vaccine.

In the U.S., despite massive vaccination against hepatitis B, the disease incidence increased by 15% in 6 years, 55 to 63 cases per hundred thousand inhabitants.

Why do you vaccinate infants against diphtheria?

Is there a diphtheria epidemic?

Did you heard in recent years some cases of diphtheria?

Serum diphtheria was discovered in 1890 by von Behring, who also took to this Nobel Prize in Medicine in 1901. Since that time the diphtheria vaccination is widespread. It was a major breakthrough in its time. Just when no one knew of antibiotics, especially penicillin to treat diphtheria.

Did you know that post-vaccination polio incidence is much higher than that of wild polio virus?

In 1976, Dr. Jonas Salk, the vaccine virus dead, testified that OPV was important, if not the sole cause of all cases of polio reported in the U.S. since 1961.

Official position recognizes the risks and inefficiencies OPV IPV:
"Disadvantages of Oral Polio Vaccine
Although OPV is safe and effective, in extremely rare Cases (approx. 1 in 2.5 Every one million doses of the vaccine, plus many unreported, inconclusive, "clean" the list) the live attenuated virus in OPV vaccines CAN cause paralysis - either in the vaccinated child, or in a close contact. Immune deficiency of the container may Be among the Causes. This risk of vaccine-Associated polio (VAPP) is well known .... . [There are countries where there is more polio vaccination, but the "natural".]

Disadvantages of inactivated Polio Vaccine

Unlike the oral vaccine, IPV confers only very little in the intestinal tract Immunity. When a person immunized with IPV is infected with wild poliovirus, the virus CAN still multiply inside the intestines and shed in stools Be - risking Continued circulation. For this reason, OPV is the vaccine of choice Wherever Outbreak of polio Needs to Be Contained, possibly in Which countries rely Exclusively on IPV for routine immunization Their programs (polio Outbreak in the Netherlands in 1992). "[That is not very effective IPV site, but let him inject children that if they have side effects ...]
(http://www.polioeradication.org/vaccines.asp)

"Today, we know that cancer induction is a phenomenon that starts from a single cell as a single functional unit of foreign DNA into host cell genome can induce malignant cell transformation. A confirmation of these truths is the discovery in 1960, the SV40 virus (Simian Virus 40) in oral polio vaccine "Sabin", prepared with live virus. It was subsequently discovered that polio vaccine "Salk" (version with inactivated virus, administered by injection) is contaminated, because the virus survives formaldehyde used for inactivation.

Researchers Sweet and Hilleman of the Merck Institute for Therapeutic Research, which made the discovery, said that all three strains of polio vaccine were found infested. SV 40 virus derived from green monkey kidney in Africa, which has grown, always, polio vaccine.

Confirmation of the oncogenes role of this virus came when the SV40 viral genome was found in various malignant tumours of adults injected with polio vaccine in infancy: mesothelioma, 3 lymphoma, non-Hodgkin's lymphoma 18, 26 brain tumours, 4, 8 osteosarcoma, 6 maxillofacial tumours.

"The Hidden virus", as they were called, have a feature that explains their names while creating destruction marked in vitro and in vivo, they are not recognized by human immune system, their structure because they needed to identify critical antigens. They determine, therefore, serious illness, train, central and peripheral nervous system, often with fatal outcomes.

The researcher said he found that they can be considered "a

biological weapon of nature", because they can wear different structural forms, but retains the ability to include in the nerve cell and destroy it.

Vaccine Act must be understood ultimately as an act of introducing foreign genetic material directly into the bloodstream. Mass vaccination campaigns have had an overwhelmingly on population, in that it led, long-term, unpredictable genetic mutations and alterations in the negative sense of the human genetic code. The link between genetic mutations and cancer in humans has been demonstrated scientifically.

The increased incidence and mortality from cancer is a reality today. On the other hand, the appearance of atypical virus, never seen before, related to contamination of vaccines, shows that, when any biological material is injected directly into the bloodstream, contamination possibilities are virtually endless and impossible to control the current science.

Did you know that although the vaccines were introduced in Europe with almost 10 years later than in the U.S., diseases for which vaccines are given only in the U.S., fell the same time and same rate and in Europe where there is still administering vaccines?

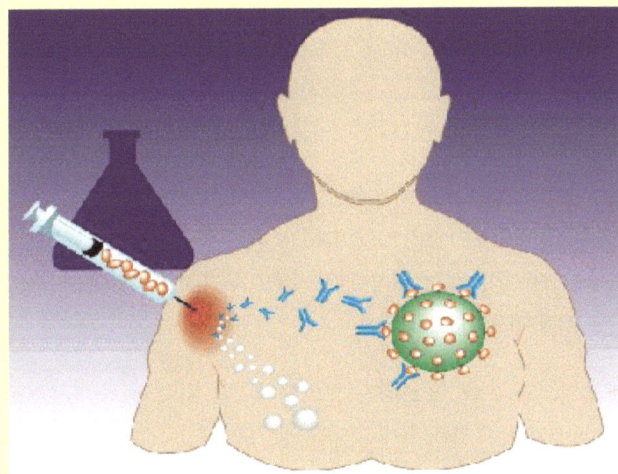

"Did you know that a child with autism may make the situation

favouring the one vaccine?"
One child leaves the hospital without a birth certificate, but with a
'Certificate of Vaccination "and made two HepB vaccines and BCG.
Plus anti- Tetanos to mother did during pregnancy. (IT IS VERY
DANGEROUS, WHEN I WAS PREGNANT I was tricked in the same
manner!!!).

These vaccines can provide immediate side effects worse than
autism, with the promise to protect children from hepatitis B and
tuberculosis. If you promise not observed (TB victims made annually
in the vaccinated population 7,000), only child remains at risk of side
effects. And if they look as in the case said the link below, then
everyone is entitled to no longer vaccinate children with no vaccine,
never. (http://iansvoice.org/default.aspx)

And about the causal link between vaccines (especially the component
that contains mercury) and autism are multiple studies have shown that
much.

There are also online, remember a few:
A. Autism: A Unique Type of Mercury poisoning
Two. Mercury on the Mind - Dr. Donald W. Miller, MD
Three. Thimerosal in Childhood Vaccines, neurodevelopment Disorders,
and Heart Disease in the U.S.
HYPERLINK "http://translate.googleusercontent.com/translate_c?
hl=en&rurl=translate.google.com&sl=ro&tl=en&u=http://www.jpands.org/vol8no1/g
eier.pdf&usg=ALkJrhiHxqzi3Y_cI72qahNkWodBEIrYTg" - MarkR. - Markram.
Geier, MD, PhD

EPI program scheme applies without informing parents about the
risks and benefits, often with pressure from doctors, without being informed
that the parents are the decision maker, without side effects or
consequences to compensate.

It seems monstrous that a baby from birth to 3 years old receives 26
vaccines, by 2 year old the toddler receives 31 vaccines, and up to year
10, the child receives 36 vaccines.

Hepatitis B vaccine is ineffective, why are boosters, which are also
inefficient, if you read the article you saw that the U.S. increase the
incidence of disease even if they are vaccinated almost entirely.

Toxicity vaccine is the worst aspect of its use need be individually customized or mass, generalized.

So, yes you can make hepatitis B even if you are vaccinated, but can be made much more serious disease than hepatitis B, as a direct result of vaccination.

The biggest lie is that this vaccine provides written final immunity. But according to the prospectus 2 to 4% of those not vaccinated do not develop antibodies, and **after a year between 1 and 8% lose their immunity**, while **you would not take the vaccine and would get it in childhood, would acquire permanent immunity naturally.**

 MMR vaccination provides immunity from claims that some minor childhood diseases **(measles, mumps, rubella),** but unnecessarily expose children vaccinated at risk of developing some serious diseases, some irreversible.

MMR vaccine can cause:

- **Autism,** *(F. Edward Yazbak, MD - "Autism: Is There a vaccine connection?" - FAAP, 1999, Avinoam Shuper, MD - "Suspected measles-mumps-rubella vaccine-related encephalitis" - Scandinavian Journal of Infectious Diseases, 15 September. 2010)*

- **Diabetes (type I), pancreatitis,** *(Harris Coulter, Ph.D. - "Childhood Vaccinations and Juvenile-onset (Type-1) Diabetes")*

- **Guillain-Barré syndrome,** *(Gros C, Spigland I. - "Guillain-Barré Syndrome Following administration of live measles vaccine" - American Journal of Medicine, March 1976, 60 (3) :441-3)*

- **Encephalitis, lymphadenopathy, febrile seizures, anaphylactic reactions, thrombocytopenic purpura, Kawasaki syndrome, erythema multiform, arthritis, meningitis, peripheral neuritis, myelitis, bronchitis, laryngitis, conjunctivitis, otites, diarrhoea, anorexia, fever, vomiting, insomnia.**

Strains of rubella, measles and mumps contain chicken embryo cells, human diploid cells, egg proteins, neomycin, lactose, sorbitol, alanine, arginine, Licinia, histidine, isoleucine, leucine, lysine, methionine, phenylalanine, proline, serine, threonine, tryptophan, tyrosine, valine, aspartic acid, cysteine, hidroxprolina.

The schedules of "routine" super - vaccinations

and about the post-vaccination new illnesses

At 24 hours after birth a new baby born took the 1st vaccine (against Hepatitis B – TOTALLY INUTILE vaccine! WE KNOW that this type of disease is taken by blood transfusion and by sexually way. It is attack to a new baby born lever in this way!)
4-7 days OF LIFE ANOTHER INUTILE vaccine (BCG)

1 MONTH, 4 vaccines (DIFTERIA, TETANUS, PERTUSSIS, OPV)

2 MONTHS, 4 vaccines (D, T, P, Hep B, OPV)
6 months, 5 vaccines (D, T, P, Hep B, OPV)
12-15 MONTHS, vaccines (R, R, A, MMR)
30-35 MONTHS, vaccines (D, T, P,).

REMARKS: The *MENINGITE C vaccine is currently not given in ROMANIA because there were registered many cases of encephalitis and autism after vaccination was given.*

The vaccine HPV given in England to girls year 8, 9 or 10 of school, ("AGAINST" CERVICAL CANCER), can give to the girls CANCER and STERILITY later.

In the spirit of compliance with relevant legislation the medical personnel shall be informing parents <u>on *non-compulsory* character of all vaccines and about all side effects damaging the health</u>.

<u>*About the triple vaccine MMR (Measles-Mumps-Rubella)*</u>

Measles vaccine is another element of the triple vaccine MMR (Measles-Mumps-Rubella), given the age of 15 months. Doctors say the vaccine is needed to prevent **measles encephalitis,** which, they argue, would occur with a frequency of 1 in 1,000 cases.

After decades of experience in cases of measles, are questioning this figure, as do many other paediatricians. Incidence of 1/1000 may be true for children living in conditions of **malnutrition** and **poverty,** but in the middle and upper classes of society, the incidence is rather **1/10,000 or 1/100,000.**

After **you scared the unlikely possibility of measles encephalitis,** sometimes your doctor will tell you about the dangers associated with measles vaccine. **Measles vaccine is associated with encephalopathy and a host of other complications such as SSPE (sub-acute scleroses pan-encephalitis), which causes solidifying material brain and is invariably fatal.**

Other sometimes fatal neurological complications associated with measles vaccine include ataxia (inability coordinate muscle movements), mental retardation, aseptic meningitis, seizures and hemiparesis (paralysis of half of the body).

Complications associated with the vaccine may be even more frightening. They include encephalitis, childhood-onset diabetes, Reye syndrome and multiple sclerosis.

I believe the risks associated with measles vaccine unacceptable, even if there was compelling evidence that the vaccine would be effective. But I'm not. The decline in disease incidence appeared long before the introduction of the vaccine. In 1958 there were approx. 800,000 cases of measles in the U.S., but in 1962, one year before a vaccine, the number of cases had dropped to 300,000.

During the next four years, while children were vaccinated with dead virus vaccine, ineffective and now abandoned, the number of cases has fallen by 300,000 since. In 1900 there were 13.3 deaths per 100,000 populations for Measles.

In 1955, before starting vaccination measles death rate had dropped to 97.7 percent, standing at value of 0.03 deaths per 100,000.

The measles illness was disappearing before the vaccine was introduced. If the numbers do not seem convincing enough, weigh out *the* following: In *1978, more than half of children who had measles in 30 U.S. states, had been vaccinated against measles. Moreover,* according to *World Health Organization,* measles chances to be contracted by those vaccinated are *15 times higher than the probability that measles will be contracted by those un- vaccinated.*

"Why, then, before all this evidence, physicians continue to vaccinate?" You ask.

Most doctors in Los Angeles responded by *injecting the vaccine to every child who has fallen into hands.* Several doctors familiar with the concept of *"slow virus",* and *immunological failure,* chose not to vaccinate their own babies.

Unlike their patients who had told no one they knew as *"slow viruses",* which are found in all vaccines and vaccine especially measles, *human tissue can hide for years and may occur later as encephalitis and multiple sclerosis.* They are also seeds and potential for development and growth of cancer later in life.

There was a Los Angeles doctor who refused to vaccinate own child seven months, said: *"I am worried about what happens to the vaccine virus, which not only offers little protection against measles, but remains hidden in the body, there acting in a way which does not know anything* ".

This concern did not stop, however, to vaccinate patients. He explained this contradictory behaviour with the comment: *"as a parent, I have the luxury to choose for my child. As a physician ... legally and professionally, I have to accept professional recommendations, as we had to do with the whole story of swine flu.* "

Measles vaccine is another element of the triple vaccine MMR (Measles-Mumps-Rubella), given the age of 15 months.

Doctors say the vaccine is needed to prevent **measles encephalitis,** which, they argue, would occur with a frequency of 1 in 1000 cases.

After decades of experience in cases of measles, are questioning this figure, as do many other paediatricians.

Incidence of 1/1000 may be true for children living in conditions of **malnutrition** and **poverty,** but in the middle and upper classes of society, the incidence is rather **1/1.0000 or 1/100.000.**

After *you scared of the unlikely possibility of measles encephalitis,* your doctor will tell you about the dangers associated with measles vaccine. *Measles vaccine is associated with encephalopathy and a host of other complications such as SSPE (sub acute sclerosis pan encephalitis), which causes the* <u>*solidifying*</u> *of the material brain and is fatal.*

Other deadly neurological complications associated with measles vaccine include ataxia (inability coordinate muscle movements), mental retardation, aseptic meningitis, seizures and hemiparesis (paralysis of half of the body). Complications associated with the vaccine may be even more frightening. They include encephalitis, childhood-onset diabetes, Reye syndrome and multiple sclerosis.

In 1958 there were approx. 800,000 cases of measles in the U.S., but in 1962, one year before a vaccine, the number of cases had dropped to 300,000.

During the next four years, while children were vaccinated with dead virus vaccine, ineffective and now abandoned, the number of cases has fallen by 300,000 since. In 1900 there were 13.3 deaths per 100,000 population for Measles.

In 1955, before starting vaccination measles death rate had dropped to 97.7 percent, standing at value of 0.03 deaths per 100,000.

The figures themselves are dramatic evidence of the fact that measles was disappearing before the vaccine was introduced.

Doctors in Los Angeles responded by *injecting the vaccine to every child who has fallen into hands.* Several doctors familiar with the concept of *"slow virus"*, and *immunological failure,* chose not to vaccinate their own babies. Unlike their patients who had told no one they knew as *"slow viruses",* which are found in all vaccines and vaccine especially measles, *human tissue can hide for years and may occur later as encephalitis and multiple sclerosis.* They are also seeds and potential for development and growth of cancer later in life.

Rubella is a benign disease of childhood that *do not require medical treatment.* Initial symptoms are *fever and mild cold sensation with pain in the neck.* We realize that's more of a cold when the characteristic rash appears on the face and scalp then spreads his arms and body.

Stains not join each other as happens in measles and usually fade and disappear in two to three days. The patient must stay in bed and be given more fluid, but no other treatment is necessary.

The only threat they present is rubella can cause damage to the foetus if a woman contracts the disease during the first three months of pregnancy.

This fear is used to justify vaccination of all children, boys and girls, as part of **MMR** vaccine (measles-mumps-rubella). The benefits of this vaccine are questionable for the same reasons exposed to mumps vaccination. No need to protect innocent children against the disease because *of vaccine side effects is unacceptable.*

They include *arthritis, arthralgia (joint pain) and polyneuritis* that causes pain, numbness or *paraesthesia* (tingling) on peripheral nerves. These symptoms are usually temporary but can last for months and can occur with a delay of up to two months after vaccination. Because the time between vaccination and adverse reactions mentioned above, *parents may not recognize the symptoms as being caused by the vaccine.*

The great danger of rubella vaccination is that, preventing illness in childhood increases the risk that women make in adolescence or adulthood disease, ie during procreation. In this way lack rubella vaccination in women of reproductive age natural immune protection that would have obtained a naturally disease.

This view is shared by many other doctors. In Connecticut a group of doctors, led by two eminent epidemiologists, have managed to eliminate rubella from the list of mandatory vaccinations. Study after study has shown that *many women vaccinated against rubella in child protective antibody not specific to adolescence.*

Other tests have shown a high failure rate of vaccination of children against measles, rubella and mumps, are administered together, either separate vaccines. Finally, the crucial question still unanswered is: *immunity from vaccine is as effective and lasts as much as obtained by contracting rubella immunity the natural way?* <u>Much of vaccinated children show lack of any immune protection in blood tests done just four to five years after vaccination.</u>

The significance of data as it is so obvious is frightening. Rubella is a dangerous disease in childhood and *provides natural immunity to those who are in childhood,* protecting them from contracting it in adulthood. Before rubella vaccination started, approx. **85%** of adults had natural immunity against rubella.

<u>**Today, because of vaccination, most women will never have natural immunity.**</u> If immunity from vaccine disappears, as expected, *they just contract rubella during pregnancy, with fatal effects on their unborn child.*

However, in a study conducted in California and published in *"Journal of the American Medical Association"*, <u>more than 90% of obstetricians-gynecologists doctors refused to be vaccinated.</u> **If doctors themselves are afraid of the vaccine, the law requires God that you and other parents to accept vaccination of your children?**

As with other infectious diseases, **whooping cough** mortality began to fall before a vaccine. The vaccine was not introduced until after 1936, but mortality began to decline steadily since 1900 and even earlier. According to Dr. Stewart, *"whooping cough mortality had declined by 80% before the introduction of the vaccine".* Share the opinion of Dr. Stewart, that the *key factor in controlling pertussis vaccine was not but improve the living conditions of potential victims.*

Common side effects of pertussis vaccine (DTP), recognized in the *"Journal of American Medical Association",* are *fever, bouts of crying,* a shock like state and local effects on the skin, such as swelling, redness and pain.

Side effects include *seizures* and *irreversible brain damage leading to mental retardation.* The vaccine was linked also and *sudden infant death syndrome.* In 1978-1979, in a widening of the vaccination program for children in Tennessee have been reported 8 cases of sudden death after DTP vaccine.

It is estimated that only 50-80% of those vaccinated presents real protection against the disease. According to the magazine *"Journal of the American Medical Association",* the number of cases of whooping cough in the U.S. is the 1000-3000 year and the number of deaths of 5-20 year.

<u>Dr. Robert S. Mendelsohn (MD)</u>: The childhood diseases linked originated in dangerous and ineffective effort done to prevent them:

MUMPS
MEASLES
RUBELLA
COUGH Whooping
DIPHTHERIA
Chickenpox
TUBERCULOSIS
Sudden infant death syndrome (SIDS)

70

POLIOMYELITIS

Not only have major doubts about vaccinations, if we were to follow my deep personal beliefs, I urge you to reject all inoculation for your child will not do that because parents of almost half of U.S. states have lost to make that choice.

Doctors, not politicians, have called for laws that force parents to vaccinate children as a prerequisite for admission to schools.

Even in these states, you could still be convinced to eliminate component paediatrician **pertussis** (whooping cough) vaccine DTP (diphtheria, tetanus, pertussis). This vaccine, which appears as the most threatening of all, is so controversial that many doctors have become anxious when they have to manage it, fearing legal malpractice actions.

Although we administered vaccines in the early years of my medical career, I became a steadfast opponent of mass inoculation because of the many dangers they pose.

In this article shall limit to my list of objections against fanatical zeal with which paediatricians injected foreign protein in your child's body without even knowing what evil can do.

There is no convincing scientific evidence that mass vaccination has led to the eradication of any disease of childhood. While it is true that some childhood diseases, once very common, the incidence decreased or disappeared after the introduction of mass vaccination, no one knows why. Rather general improvement of living conditions may be the reason.

If vaccination was the reason of the disappearance of these diseases in the U.S., we can **ask why they disappeared simultaneously in Europe, where mass vaccination is not practised.**

It is believed that the Salk polio vaccine led to stopping the epidemic of polio that affected American children in 1940 and 1950.

If so, why stop polio epidemic also in Europe, where polio vaccine was not used extensively? An even more relevant question is: **of the Sabin vaccine virus is still given to children when Dr. Jonas Salk, who prepared the first polio vaccine in the world, shows that Sabin vaccine strain is currently causing most cases of polio in children?**

Further vaccination forced the children with this vaccine is an irrational medical practice that confirms my opinion that doctors consistently repeated mistakes. The situation is identical **stubbornness medical world to give up vaccination vaccine to 3 decades after the disappearance of the disease, when the vaccine remained the only source of contamination and death from smallpox.**

Think about this! **For 30 years, children have died of smallpox vaccine, though no longer threatened by natural disease.**

There are significant risks associated with each vaccine and numerous contraindications that make vaccines to be risky for your children

However, doctors administer them routinely, usually without warning parents about the risks and without **to investigate whether these vaccines are not initially contraindicated for a child. No child would be vaccinated initially to investigate the existence and possible contraindications.**

However, the small army of children are lined up in clinics to get shot in the arm, without their parents to ask any questions!

While many short-term side effects after vaccination is known (but rarely explained), no one knows the long term consequences of injecting foreign proteins the human body in your child's body Even more shocking is that no one makes no a coherent effort to learn.

There is growing suspicion that immunization against relatively harmless childhood diseases is responsible for the dramatic increase in autoimmune diseases, growth occurs after the introduction of mass vaccination of children.

It's the dreaded disease, like *leukaemia, cancer, rheumatoid arthritis, multiple sclerosis, Lou Gehrig's disease, lupus erythematosus and Guillain-Barre syndrome.*

An autoimmune disease can be simply defined as a situation in which the body's defence mechanisms cannot distinguish between foreign invaders and their tissues and, consequently, destroy their own structures.

I gave it the measles mumps and cancer and leukaemia? I have highlighted these problems because **Your paediatrician probably will not prevent them. Forum on the American Academy of Paediatrics**

(AAP) in 1982 he proposed a resolution that would have provided information to parents about the risks and benefits of vaccination.

Resolution urging that "to make known in simple language understandable to any rational parent, risks and benefits of routine vaccines, diseases against which the vaccine risks and management of the most common adverse reactions".

It seems that doctors did not consider that **a "reasonable parent"** is entitled to this type of information that **rejected the resolution!**

Bitter controversy about vaccinations, taken within the medical profession has not escaped media attention. A number of increasingly more parents refuse to vaccinate their children, supporting legal sanctions accordingly.

Parents whose children have suffered irreversible damage after vaccination no longer resign to the situation and initiates legal action against vaccine manufacturers or doctors who administered the vaccine.

The existence of mandatory vaccinations cause patients who otherwise would have no reason to go to the paediatrician, were required to come only periodically for vaccination, so vaccination became very usually in the paediatric practice.

Therefore, paediatricians will continue to the death to defend the concept of compulsory vaccination.

My PERSONAL COMMENT:

*In the communist regime in **Romania,** nobody asked about parents consent to vaccinate a child. Millions of children were vaccinated against their will and against their parents will. Most of parents they did not know at that time that the vaccines are very dangerous for health. Nobody told them about the poisons from vaccines.*

I was vaccinated compulsory in the school when I was 7 and 9 years old with multiple vaccines.

I had very easily in my entire life respiratory disease-causing from vaccines, allergies, autoimmune disease and when I was 29 years old I was paralysed 4 weeks all body and I was almost to die because of a myelo -poli- radiculo- nevrites illness caused by polio vaccine. That malefic virus was living in my spinal liquid according to the laboratory tests from hospital and it was alive after more than twenty years !

Criminally infected children with AIDS in Romania orphanages by immunization campaigns after 1989

HOW FAR AWAY the malefic evil & masonic leaders who are ruling this world they can go ? As information about big pharmaceutical companies from Western Europe, it has been conducting a program of HIV infection of a few thousands of innocent children in ROMANIA'S orphanages (by vaccinations with live AIDS virus) from the cradle to study AIDS and find remedy. Nowadays statistics are much more bigger.

This program was launched in the years 1987-1990 and involved a number of researchers in immunology from WESTERN EUROPE. It was very easy to infect pure innocent children with no parents from ROMANIA...

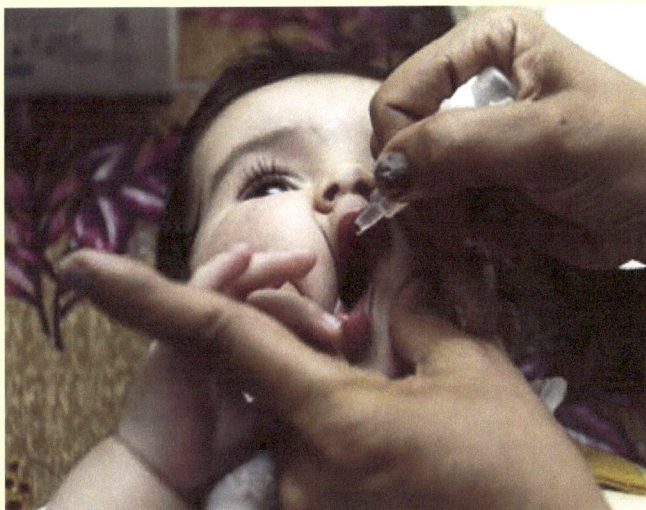

 Nobody ask about them , they did not have parents to take care of them or to ask questions or   even to start court trial between state and who came with HUNDRED OF TRUCKS "HELP" for ROMANIA" ...

 That transports included thousands of shots of vaccines deliberately with <u>alive viruses</u> to kill by vaccination ROMANIA'S children.

<u>M</u>ore than half of children with AIDS across the globe are Romanians! How is this possible given that the rate of spread of the disease in Romania in adults is much lower? Regarding the situation in Romania there are *some disturbing evidence on deliberate HIV infection of children.*

This was achieved during vaccination campaigns against hepatitis B. It is also highly significant that although hepatitis B vaccine has not been sufficiently tested and although, in fact, the vaccination campaign costs a lot (reason why the French Health Ministry refused the vaccination campaign) but the Ministry of Health of Romania with the direct involvement of former minister Iulian Mincu sponsored by Rotary Club (which is a satellite of world freemasonry) imposed free and compulsory vaccination of children in Romania (again, given that the vaccine has not been sufficiently tested).

 The Government Decree No. 41.566 of 22 August 1995 on vaccinating children against hepatitis B developed under the national immunization stated: "In Romania, HBV infection is prevalent from the first year of life. The porting rate it was estimated at 4.9% in children aged 6-11 months.

World Health Organization recommends universal vaccination integration of newborns in national vaccination programs until 1995 in countries where HBV porting rate is at least 8% and in all countries by the year 1997 (...) Vaccination against hepatitis B is compulsory for all children born since 10/01/1995 ".
The former Health Minister Iulian Mincu was slow to realize this so controversial vaccinations. We naturally ask the question why?

An Italian journalist claims to have evidence to prove intentional HIV infection of Romanian children. Story published by "Event Day" in Romania that many children were infected with HIV virus that causes AIDS, has been rattled in Italy.

The Italian journalist Mino Damato said that he has clear evidence about at least six cases of children infected with HIV in this way.

Mr Damato, which in Italy has a strong reputation as a serious and independent television journalist, has often been in Romania since 1989. He raised one million dollars for children with AIDS, fund managed by the foundation he runs, "Bambini in Emergenza".

(HOWEVER, a part of the money raised by the Italian association were used to build a new pavilion for children with AIDS at the hospital "Victor Babes" in Bucharest. Mr Damato sent an appeal to the government in Bucharest, seeking to shed light on this tragedy, to be identified and punished those responsible for these crimes. (Source : PAOLO GIANFELICI, "Event Day" - 2/25/1997, no. 1418)

My personal comment : The Italian journalist efforts are irrelevant to help indeed those Romanian children... In that new hospitals built with the donation money, the HIV deliberately infected children are still used by the Romanian doctors as laboratory ""mice"" to test new medicines against AIDS.

A new confirmation : the children in Romania

were contaminated with HIV intentionally

Surprising discovery from Iasi city specialists doctors : AIDS was transmitted intentionally, in cradles of children in Romania, from a single source. It confirms the hypothesis infected orphans for research.

Laboratory of Virology Iasi specialists of the University of Medicine and Pharmacy "Grigore T. Popa", Iasi, in collaboration with Institute experts "Pasteur" in Paris, managed to pool after five years of research, the results of cases HIV-AIDS in children registered in Romania.

The author is *Dr. Cristian Apetrei* research, doctoral student at the "Pasteur" and professor doctor at the Medicine University of Iasi. The results confirmed the first time that HIV with infected children was a swing from a single source.

The hypothesis of deliberate HIV infection in Romanian children orphanages in order to do research and find the antidote to the disease is confirmed by scientific research. **(The source is the prof. doctor CRISTIAN APETREI).**

HIV infection does not come from hospital

Dr. Cristian Apetrei said about an unequivocal conclusion: "Our research confirms the responsibility of subtype F in producing an epidemic of HIV infection in children in Romania. Isolation of a unique subtype of all the historical provinces of the country to demonstrate the unitary character of the epidemic and confirms the description of the risk group of children in care units. Structural similarity between different isolates suggests the possibility of evolution from a single source epidemic "

Intentionally infected blood was distributed in areas of ROMANIA

The Discovery of doctors is of utmost importance! It proves that the same source of infection has not occurred by transfusion, as both donors and blood supply structures of the health system and was not centralized, even before 1989. "This source remains obscure, if we consider that paediatric health system is organized at regional level, and blood transfusion from the same source is distributed throughout the country," mentions the article signed by the Romanian Medicine Professor Doctor MD, Cristian Apetrei.

The Romanian health system is absolved of guilt

Research are supported by statistics of HIV cases registered in Romania. In Romania country there are, according to World Health Organization, over 50% of children infected with HIV in the world.

 In addition, the material also points out that type of virus found in adults, which are actually visible, infected from multiple sources, are totally different than the types of material recorded in children from orphanages (with no parents).

In this case, in Romania, infection in hospitalized children in orphanages is more "strange" because, even in neighbouring countries, which had similar health care systems, in children or in adults, the incidence of epidemic was smaller.

A terrifying scenario: Children as guinea pigs

Updated data on HIV infection in Romania in February 1997, are as follows: 3,121 people with HIV and 85% children and 4,446 people with AIDS, of which 4,005 CHILDREN. Official data and recent findings confirm the hypothesis supported by some statements by doctors, subject anonymity.

According to them, in our country ROMANIA has been conducting a program of HIV infection of children from the cradle to study AIDS and find remedy.

This program was launched in the years 1987-1988 and involved a large number of doctors in immunology. *(source : Iulian Chifu, "The Event Day" , ROMANIA - 1997).*

Everyone knows that AIDS was artificially created in USA laboratories...But WHY they spread this HIV viruses between innocent children from Romanian orphanages?

What about the 2013 statistics of infected HIV children and adults in Romania ? GOD knows! There are top-secret files and the Romanian Medical authorities give no information to the public and journalists!

The mercury from vaccines

and the autism disease

WASHINGTON, DC - A new study published in *"Journal of the Neurological Sciences'* official journal of the *World Federation of Neurology,* which is an NGO affiliated with the World Health Organization, associated mercury in vaccines (Thiomersal) with autism and other disorders of neurological development. *(HA Young, Geier DA, Geier MR.* **Thimerosal Exposure in Infants and neuro- development Disorders:** *An Assessment of Computerized medical records in the Vaccine Safety datalink. J Neurol Sci. 2008 May 14. Full article is available at: http://www.pharmalot.com/wp-content/uploads/2008/05/thimerosal-vaccine- study.pdf)*

This study is six years of efforts by independent researchers access to data to be kept secret in the Vaccine Safety data link (VSD) by the U.S. Centres for disease prevention and the control (CDC famous). In 2003 the Governmental Committee for Reform of the U.S. House of Representatives called for "... access for independent researchers to the database" Vaccine Safety data link "because of the need to study and independent validation of CDC studies regarding exposure of children to mercury contained in vaccines and research links it with autism.

The irony is that only a few independent researchers have had the right to access this level so restrictive VSD data bank, despite the VSD project is funded by hundreds of millions of taxpayer dollars.

The study, led by Dr. Heather Young, Ph.D., professor of epidemiology at the University of George Washington and public health services, examined records held by the CDC vaccination **of 278,624 children** born between **1990-1996.** In this study we calculated average mercury exposure children have supported routine vaccination with vaccines containing thiomersal, depending on year of birth, and that vaccination performed in infancy. After calculating average mercury exposure by year of birth, the study estimated the prevalence of various medical diagnoses established for children in each year examined.

Sampled rate of autism and other disorders of neurological development was correlated with average mercury exposure children: increase / decrease the level of mercury exposure of children vaccinated with vaccines containing thiomersal routine shows the trend of increasing / decreasing the rate of diagnosis question. By contrast, medical results not supposed to be related to mercury, not correlated with the average level of mercury exposure due to vaccines Thiomersal.

With different specific neurological development disorders (autism, autistic spectrum disorders, emotional disturbance, attention deficit and hyperactivity and learning difficulties) the overall risk of developing autism and neurological disorders observed was significantly higher (between 2 up to 6 times) for an exposure of 100 micrograms of mercury. Autism itself, the overall risk was 2.5 times higher at 100 micrograms of mercury exposure.

The mercury in vaccines gives:

- *Action allergic*

- *Hyperactivity syndrome (ADHD)*

- *Autism*

- *Studies show link between mercury and autism*

Because they contain substances, vaccines intoxicate the body, with serious consequences over time. If vaccines were considered over time, the reputation they have acquired a true "holy cow", good milking, would not have been possible *prolonged use of neuro- toxine substances used as preservatives such as mercury, without need.* Why? Just because it has always been and perhaps because no one questioned the "safety" in preparations with a historical past so famous. (The medical manual "Lob der Krankheit" Bert Ehgartner, 2008, p 175).

Mercury was first used by the physician Girolamo Fracastoro of Verona - fellow of the German doctor Paracelsius for the treatment of syphilis. Treatment was awful, patients had severe pain. Most died of syphilis or remained with neurological illness (increased tremor, etc.). *Fracastoro himself, in 1546, draws attention to the danger of mercury.*

Until the twentieth century, when it is discovered antibiotics, mercury remains the basic treatment of syphilis treatment.

The use of mercury in vaccines is a composition usually from twentieth century: in 1930 U.S. pharmaceutical company Eli Lilly for the first time *thiomersal* used to manufacture diphtheria vaccine. A percentage of 49.6% of the substance containing organic mercury, neuro- toxic. At that time vaccines were not individualized, but were kept in larger container, where the doctor was used as needed, then still stored in the refrigerator. So I needed a preservative.

Either mercury's toxicity to bacteria protect vaccine. Has done so because in 1928, immediately after vaccination, 11 children died. Although it was clear to those of Eli Lilly and new preservative that can be dangerous for the body, continued to believe that a small dose of mercury could be toxic to the nervous system.

This error has led to decades for mercury as a preservative for many vaccines. Only vaccines that contain live viruses such as polio and measles vaccines have no mercury, because it would destroy viruses.

During this time have heard many voices warn of the danger posed by mercury in vaccines, is a real nerve poison. Only in the mid-90s, the U.S. Departments of Health, following studies on the effect of mercury on the body, finds that the real problem of Thiomersal upon human health. As the *number of vaccines has tripled between 1980-2000, had risen because of the dose of mercury used in their preparation* .

A 5 kg baby may receive a higher dose of 34 micrograms of mercury, according to EPA and WHO's 159 micrograms (more "lenient"). An infant receiving all prescribed vaccines in the first 14 weeks of age, body collects an amount of 187.5 micrograms of mercury.

Or the poisoning of the body takes place just at the time the baby's nervous system develops, otherwise very sensitive at this stage.

The greatest danger was found in children born prematurely, weighing less than normal. One paper shows that *it is enough antihepatite B vaccine, given a small infant exceeds 10 times the dose of mercury accepted by EPA. (GV Stajich et al. "Iatrogenic exposure to mercury after Hepatitis B vaccination in pre term children", J . Pediatr 2000, 136: 679-81.)*

The U.S. officials have still not concluded correctly that should be ruled out mercury from all vaccines for infants.

Therefore, only in 2001, began to appear on the market vaccines for infants, without containing thiomersal (mercury). HOWEVER , THE VACCINES ARE VERY DANGEROUS, TOO.

The hardest part this was done with influenza vaccines. But even today can produce vaccines with thiomersal, particularly those with longer term use.

Following the recommendations of WHO's express, longer term use manufactured vaccines containing thiomersal. (Ibid, p 179, Lob der K.)

b) Action of Thiomersal:

Allergic action: all vaccines containing thiomersal cause allergic reactions. The allergy vaccine used recently that "sensitized almost whole of Austria" (Wolfgang Maurer, Wien), was not against *borreliosis caused by tick bite.*

Hyperactivity syndrome (ADHD)

The scientists made the connection between thiomersal and ADHD. Cases occurring far exceed those of autism. Approximately *5% of babies born / year* suffer from this syndrome, called in Germany, "Zappelphilipps" and 1-2 children in a class have the syndrome. The situation is even worse *in the U.S. where 9% of children aged between 8 and 15 years suffering from ADHD. "(TE* Froehlich et al. 'Prevalence, recognition and Treatment of Attention - Deficit / Hyperactivity Disorder in a national sample of U.S. children", Paediatrician Med. 2007; 161 (9) :857-864.) 1/3 of these children (2, 4 million) requires drugs and other third take medication "as needed". Psychologists treat these children through "behavioural therapies".

Autism

There was a link between high doses of mercury in infants and soaring cases of neurological disorders, especially autism. When in 1943, psychiatrist Leo Kanner at Johns Hopkins Hospital in Baltimore, described the first cases of autism in children, Thiomersalul was already used a decade as a preservative in vaccine production. (Ibid., p 180-181), but not yet studied the toxicity of nerve.

This is why Leo Kanner believed that autism is caused mainly by animal proteins in vaccines. Then it will show that not only these foreign proteins bearing "fault" but toxic substances like mercury and aluminium in vaccines are able to cause autism in children. It is true that in all children with autism are, as for those with allergies or autoimmune disease, a genetic substrate, a predisposition to these diseases. But not much longer seeks the cause of autism to a "defective gene". *It takes an "external factors" (triggers) that cause disease.*

Studies show that the "explosion" of autism cases in the U.S. occurred between 1987 - 1992, when new vaccines were introduced in infants, with a mercury content of three times. "(Newschaffer CJ et al. National autism prevalence trends from United States special education data ", Paediatrics 2005, 115: 277-282).

The relation between

mercury from vaccines and autism

It appeared more and more studies on the toxic effects of mercury on the nervous system of children. Scientists have asked parents "mop" of babies to perform toxicological studies. (Ibid, p 183).

What was found was to start a paradox for all: *the hair amount of mercury in children was 8 times higher than in those with autism!* (AS Holmes et al. "Reduced levels of mercury in first baby haircuts of autistic children", International Journal of Toxicology 2003 22: 277-285).

The autism was more serious, the amount of mercury in hair was lower.

This demonstrates that children with autism can not excrete mercury from the body, either by urine or hair. Instead it accumulates in the body. A number of studies show that children with autism have a much higher concentration of heavy metals in the body than the healthy. (R. Nataf et al. 'Porphyritic in childhood autistic disorder: Implications for Environmental Toxicity, "Toxicology and Applied Pharmacology 2006; 214:99-108).

Managing children with autism medication which removes heavy metals, mercury was detected immediately. The mercury from urine was up to 6 times higher in children with autism compared to healthy children studied.

This is the Thiomersal content in vaccines. (Bradstreet J et al. "A case - control study of mercury burden in children with autism spectrum Disorders", Journal of American Physicians and Surgeons 2003 2003, 8: 76-79).

 Martha **Herbert,** specialist in child neurology at Harvard University sought an explanation. Studying the brains of these children suffering from autism, found that their weight is much higher than normal.

This may be an excess of heavy metals which in turn causes inflammation and brain infections.

Is there a real epidemic of autism in the U.S.A. Even the CDC (Center for Disease Control in the U.S.) made a statistic: in the '70s to record 1-2 cases per 10 000 children at the turn of the millennium, one child in 166 per 10 000 suffers from autism. Boys are more frequently affected: one in 60, while girls rarely: one of 250.

While officials recognize the seriousness of the situation, they still see the exact cause is unknown and that only mercury in vaccines could be responsible for this because peoples can ingest this metal in various foods (eggs, fish) in a quantity greater than exists in vaccines, but ignore that is a very big difference between the mercury content of foods and vaccines.

Thomas Burbacher, a professor at the University of Washington, Seattle, specializing in Labor and Environmental Medicine, has done research on apes, studying the effect of dietary mercury in vaccines and the nervous system. **Mercury from thiomersal in vaccines appears in the form of ethyl-mercury and in food-which contains-mercury as methyl-mercury.**

This important aspect was not studied for decades, because they believe that mercury in vaccines is rapidly cleared from the body. What went wrong? Elimination of blood does not mean removal from the body. Heavy metals in the blood disappear but they can still exists inside the organ!

Professor Thomas Burbacher has seen that ethyl-mercury in vaccines is no longer found in the blood after 8.5 days of the shot instead of methyl-mercury in the blood which disappears later, only after 21.5 days. *It says that indeed mercury in vaccines is eliminated faster than the food.* But the way out for mercury in the two cases was different: **mercury in food (methyl-mercury) is eliminated in the faeces and bile predominant and is found in the brain only a 10% as non -organic mercury (less toxic).**

Mercury in vaccines (ethyl mercury) is detected as follows: one part urine and blood goes elsewhere in the brain, transformed into metallic mercury in a 71% (very toxic!) It also noted that eliminating mercury metal in the brain is several times slower than blood. This is why the toxic mercury is stored in the brain. (Burbacher TM - Comparison of blood and brain mercury levels in infant monkeys Exposed to methyl-mercury or Vaccines containing thiomersal" Environmental Health Perspectives - published online 21. April 2005).

Institute of Medicine of the U.S. - one of the highest courts of Health - admitted a possible link to order "biological" between mercury in vaccines and neurological disorders. *(Institute of Medicine "Immunization Safety Review - Thimerosal - Containing Vaccines and Neurological Developmental Disorders", The National Academy of Sciences 2001).* But three years later experts believe that there is no such link and no longer requires further studies.

Dr. Thomas Burbacher simply feel that this attitude is strange, given that almost no known toxic effects of Thiomersalului on-stage nervous system development and maturation. It is however a toxic substance that is injected millions of infants in all the countries. He ends his article thus: "Methyl-mercury is not the correct reference substance which can be studied and known toxic effects of mercury on the human nervous system (...)." (Ibid, p 187).

Unfortunately, such voices have remained in the minority. Most epidemiological studies in this respect have been banned in Denmark since 1992. (KM Madsen - 'Thiomersal and the occurrence of autism: Negative Ecological Evidence from Danish Population-based data ", Pediatrics 2003, 112: 604-606).

After the discovery was made public a routine check out revealed that the excess of mercury in infants vaccinated with thiomersal- type of mercury.

The officials finally responded and provided enough money to study the vaccinated children and effects of the years of vaccinations.

Burbacher's studies, which already dates from 2005, are taken into account just now.

As a result, the WHO henceforth prohibits the use of thiomersal in vaccine production site, but only in industrialized countries, while in sub-developed countries it further recommends ... (!!!) (ibid, p 189).

 W.H.O.'s position was not a very easy. On the one hand, the number of associations of parents of autistic children who accused the vaccine manufacturers for their fatal mistakes (and it was understandable that it will be related to processes large amounts imminent), and on the other pharmaceutical industry threatened to will withdraw all of the production of vaccines that will be protected by law.

For the Medical Science it was impossible to go back to the past and to recognize that medicine was wrong as long ... A new study about the link between mercury and nerve disorders should also be avoided. So the compromise is to produce the vaccines with thiomersal, but only for some countries (not very important, but they can pay very big money to buy the poisoning vaccines!... (Ibid, p 191-192).

Aluminium in vaccines :

the dirty "little" secret of immunology

If mercury was known for certain that "because of its toxicity was used as a preservative in vaccines and in case of contamination by bacteria or fungi from the beginning had to destroy them, the same can said that *aluminium is "a heavy metal found in two thirds of all vaccines on the market and the effect that no one knows practically nothing, but without the vaccine simply does not work."* ("Lob der Krankheit" Bert Ehgartner, 2008, pp. 192-193). Charles Janeway Jr., Immunology at Yale University in New Haven, calls aluminium for these reasons as "dirty little secret" of immunology. (*Charles Janeway Jr., "Approaching the Asymptote" Evolution and revolution in immunology ", 1989 54 , 1: 1-13);*

Using *of aluminium as an adjuvant (from* the Latin "adjuvare" = support) in vaccines, has a history as long as mercury is. Already in 1931 Alexander Thomas Glenny has been published his discovery about the *new diphtheria vaccine for using aluminium as an adjutant.* Although it's been so long since this toxic metal used to make vaccines, not practical knowledge of the mechanism of action (Lob der Krankheit, p 193);

- In 2006 first appears an article written by Scottish immunologist James M. Brewer, "(How) do aluminium adjutants work-?", Immunology Letters 2006; 102:10-15). In the article he expresses surprise that, **although aluminium is used for over 70 years despite it does** _not know anything about the chemical reaction between it and the_ _antigen in vaccines and no studies on the biological effect of aluminium in the body._ It's just that aluminium increases the body's immune response to vaccine antigen. This is achieved through several mechanisms.

First link of adjuvant and antigen is blocked in this way the effect of deposit. From this antigen is released slowly and thus a greater number of immune cells in contact with the antigen, the immune response is larger (by macrophages, dendrites cells and lymphocytes).

The role of adjutant use is to amplify the immune response against the antigen without inducing an immune reaction but also against himself.

Then adjutant should be removed from the body. So here is the theory ... But experience shows that it have used almost exclusively inorganic salts, heavy soluble, hard releasing antigen.

Most common are aluminium salts as aluminium phosphate and aluminium hydroxide. The advantage of aluminium is that it favours a high production of antibodies, so immune serum (specific antibody-forming), but not cellular immunity (general involving T type of lymphocytes).

There are vaccines that do not require adjutants, such as alive vaccines *(measles, etc.),* because they have enough "power ?" to induce immunity. Live viruses have got therefore their own adjutants. The "killed virus" vaccines usually do not require adjutants, but can cause sufficient immunity. However, vaccines that contain only "particles of bacteria" or "antigenic surface protein", cannot induce sufficient immunity and requires the use of adjutants, aluminium salts.

- Aluminium salts that _cause infections at the injection site_ it is a signal to the immune system;

  – - Our immune system sometimes reacts in a totally unexpected, as it did not want immunologists. _It is known that aluminium often causes allergic reactions and_ _even autoimmune diseases._ Not be neglected local reactions caused by aluminium, is sometimes very difficult to cure. Aluminium salts dissolve hard, remaining a long time causing local irritation at the injection site pain.

  – However immunologists have not found out better alternative to aluminium. An alternative would be just another obstacle ... mercury. Therefore official institutions prefer not to studies to discover the true effects of aluminium in the body. Vaccine manufacturers are even less interested to initiate such studies, and damaging the sale of so profitable.

– - *Yehuda Shoenfeld from Autoimmune Disease Centre at the University of Tel Aviv* published a series of works about the causes of these diseases. A Congress was held in 2006, which they were discussed the potential risks of vaccines. He outlined how those vaccines can cause self-harm and consequently autoimmune diseases.

– It is a mechanism called "molecular mimicry" like antigen molecules at the surface may be identical with the body's own molecules.

It is a problem when our immune system reacts and attacks its own cells. So develop autoimmune disease.

You got in action and all that tricks the immune system and directs immune cells to death some proteins of the body and not on the surface of antigens in vaccines.

There is a danger that immune cells react against their own cells. A concrete example: a group of researchers from the University Research Vancouver in Canada studied the effect of vaccine adjutants in mice. The study was performed particularly to search for causes of disease then called "Gulf War Syndrome", they had thousands of soldiers who fought in the War (1990-1991).

The uranium weapons were not used to war or nerve gas in Iraq, but very sophisticated vaccination program applied these soldiers before they leave the Gulf. One of the evidence was a Syndrome of both the soldiers who left the Gulf and those who have never gone to war left behind, but all of them were vaccinated.

The worst symptoms came up in the nerves, with severe neuromuscular damage (French soldiers, not treated with such vaccines have not suffered from the Gulf War syndrome).

The authors noted *that "aluminium hydroxide caused gait and behaviour were seen in the presence of large numbers of neurons are in a stage prior to death),in different regions of the central nervous system and a large number of motor neurons were destroyed in spinal cord.* "(Ibid, p 198).

Canadian scientists presented on this occasion and many other studies done on humans and animals showing the disastrous effects of aluminium salts in human health by enabling not only the nerve disease, but also various autoimmune diseases and allergies.

They particularly warned of the danger of aluminium in vaccines for infants: "the continued use of aluminium adjutants with different vaccines (hepatitis A and B, DTP = diphtheria, tetanus, pertussis, etc..), May have serious health for a long time.

So there will be no safety studies on vaccines for a long period. *To study effects on the nervous system will be impossible, because many of those vaccinated will be sick at that time.... "Put the inevitable question of whether the risk of vaccines is not much higher than the disease to be prevented. Unfortunately, say Canadian scientists have not received any request for such studies related to vaccine manufacturers or pharmaceutical companies. Their studies were funded by two private research firms in Canada "/-*

– **- The existence of enormous quantities of salt of mercury (thimerosal) in** vaccines, the amount declared by the producers themselves, expressed in units unfit to appear negligible (0.01% they say, you should express mercury "per share billion "(ppb), drive the maximum concentration of 2 ppb in drinking water and a dose of vaccine is the amount of 100,000 ppb (equivalent of 0.01%)).

— When a waste has more than 200 ppb mercury is considered toxic waste and require special disposal, storage and transport, and if a vaccine the mercury- thimerosal has got 100,000 ppb (about 50,000 ppb mercury) seem normal to inject in our children body?

— <u>Clinical effects of chronic mercury poisoning the cumulative effect of mercury through vaccines</u>

- Statistical correlation between mercury in vaccines and autism incidence (* first case of autism described in 1932, mercury in vaccines was introduced in 1931, * after the introduction of widely 60-70 years incidence of autism has increased from one case to one hundred thousands of people, from one case to 150 people in 2005 who refused vaccination * communities have no cases of illness of autism (the 20,000 non-vaccinated Amish, there is no autism.)

- Medical evidence (biochemical and clinical) shows that autism is a form of mercury that occurs in response to many children exposed to mercury vaccine.

— - Treatment with mercury shows lower mercury in tissue, increasing the excretion of mercury, dramatic improvements neuro- psychological condition of the patient (a case shows that, after 6 months treatment to eliminate the mercury from the body, the child began to speak again).

Vaccines cause infant mortality in children

Medical Study

A shocking study recently published in a prestigious medical journal has found a direct statistical link between the number of vaccine doses administered and the infant mortality rate in the developed world. Inoculation study suggests that the number of medical authorities imposed forced child actually has a negative impact on health. The number of doses of vaccine is growing - especially in the United States, which administers most vaccines and have, also, the highest number of infant deaths.

The study, titled "Regression infant mortality rate to the number of vaccine doses required: no biochemical or synergistic toxicity" (" Against Infant Mortality rates regressed number of vaccine doses routinely given: Is There a biochemical or Synergistic Toxicity? "), the was led by Neil Z. Miller and Gary S. Goldman and published in the prestigious journal "Human and Experimental Toxicology" (Human and Experimental Toxicology Journal), which is indexed in the National Library of Medicine.

The study states that "the average linear regression analysis of infant mortality rate demonstrated a significant statistical correlation between high number of doses of vaccine and child mortality You can see how similar are the two lists, seven of the most developed 10 countries with the lowest infant mortality rates appear in the top 10 countries that administered the vaccines less.

Note, in addition, in this table, as the two countries which vaccinate the least civilized children (Japan and Sweden) are also in the top of the column with the lowest infant mortality rates, while the States United is the opposite: with most vaccines given to children (26 before the age of one year), are the first in infant mortality (6.22 deaths per 1,000 live births).

Note also that the U.S. is ahead of Cuba or Slovenia in infant mortality, while spending more on medical care compared to these two countries.

The study clearly illustrates that **developed countries that manage fewer vaccines have lower infant mortality rates,** and suggests a direct statistical link between infant deaths and side effects of vaccination.

In As one of the richest people on Earth, Bill Gates often meets secretly with other billionaires to discuss ways to reduce world population. One of such meetings took place on May 5, 2009.

The vaccinations are linked to pharmaceutical profits rather than protect human health.

[1] http://www.prisonplanet.com/bill-gates-use-vaccines-to-lower-population.html
[2] http://www.gatesfoundation.org/vaccines/Pages/default.aspx
[3] http://www.prisonplanet.com/the-real-story-behind-bill-gates-and-death-panels.html
[4] http://www.timesonline.co.uk/tol/news/world/us_and_americas/article6350303.ece

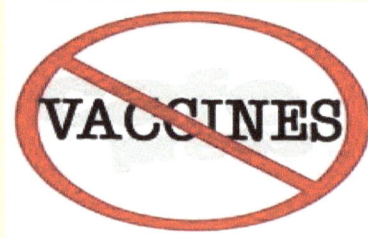

Tetanus vaccine

Tetanus is a disease caused by a bacterium called *Clostridium tetanus,* which enters the body in the wound. The bacteria can form spores that are very resistant in the environment, especially in the soil and animal droppings (especially horses).

The easiest is by biting infected wounds, burns, bites and wounds especially foreign body: wood, glass, metal. (Behrman 1999). *A bleeding wound, well oxygenated, it will never contain tetanus toxin. It is found only in anaerobic conditions (without oxygen environments).* With the advent of modern vehicles in cities, which took place horse carriages, there is less infection with this bacillus.

 Infection is favoured by diseases such as diabetes and atherosclerosis (ATS), when patients have poor circulation. Bacteria multiply very well in conditions of poor circulation, lack of oxygen.

Bacillus poison called tetanus toxin has an affinity for the nervous system. It spreads along nerves and reach central nervous system (CNS).

Depending on how close it is nerves or spinal injury, disease is reached within 4 days - 2 weeks. Tetanus toxin affects motor activity (muscle), leading to generalized muscle contractions and very painful, with preservation of consciousness.

 The most dangerous are respiratory muscle contraction. Emergency treatment is. Mortality was higher in the past.

Since 1980, never recorded no means fatal to children in Germany. Even the elderly, we see a significant decrease in fatal cases, the cause is probably getting smaller spread of bacteria (the mechanization of agriculture, modernization of transport, etc.). *Since 2001 is not considered a disease to be reported in obligatorily.*

90

In the 3rd world countries, including in ROMANIA, the W.H.O. (World Health Organization), "make sure" there are still many cases of tetanus deaths, therefore, recommended to vaccinate pregnant women who transmitted the 6 months post-partum protection to their children???. (W.H.O. study 2000).

Tetanus is considered a disease of civilization that you, being more common in underdeveloped countries. In a study of 89 non-vaccinated people in Mali, found that nearly half of them had a reliable protection against tetanus, with enough antibodies and baby in case of pregnancy. (Ehrengut, 1983).

It is possible that poor food and unsanitary conditions of children lead to a common infection causing bacteria in the intestines an effective defence by antibody formation.

Young children always go to mouth objects and this can be put in contact with this bacteria and antibodies but since an early age.

Even those non-vaccinated, tetanus can be prevented if the wound is treated immediately and properly disinfected. The disease, including less developed countries, 93% of young patients with disease of moderate can be cured with conventional treatment (antibiotics: penicillin and metronidazole).

The famous German surgeon, Professor Hackethal, writes about this vaccine for 30 years tried to avoid it if open wounds.

Explaining what possible risk patients may be exposed after the vaccine, almost none left never vaccinated and yet, had no case of tetanus. (Dr.med G . Buchwald, *Impfen. Das Geschäft mit der Angst,* 2008, s.118-119)

<u>Tetanus vaccine</u> contains *tetanus toxin, with a mortality rate 50 times higher* than natural, but formalin inactivated.

Infants have got a <u>very small</u> risk of infection with the bacterium that causes tetanus. *Through DTP (administered 4 times by the age of 12 months) are introduced into infant body toxin tetanus toxin with diphtheria, pertussis antigen and adjutant allergy - aluminium hydroxide ALOH3 - which can cause allergies, autoimmune diseases, neurological diseases or even sudden death. (by Viera* Scheibner, 2000).

- About the *Aluminium hydroxide:*

With vaccines in early infancy, babies take *2.4 milligrams of aluminium* given *stored in the bone marrow, nervous system, kidneys and muscles. (Keith 2000).* At a 6 kg infant receiving only <u>*hexa-vaccines (includes DTP), aluminium is exceeded dose limits stipulated by the "American Society for Clinical Nutrition" 60 times.*</u> Some children can not remove aluminium from the body. (Bradstreet 2004). In Romania, DTP vaccine, which is found in aluminium hydroxide, administered 4 times by the age of one year.

Aluminium causes infections in the muscles and lymph nodes to abscess formation. Sometimes persist for years itching of the nodules remaining small and red.

<u>*Neurological effects*</u> are the most feared: aluminium is transported through the nervous system of substances which cause allergic and toxic reactions. (Redhead 1992).

Aluminium caused nerve disorders are: behavioural disorders, drowsiness, depression, memory problems. The high concentration of aluminium will cause the destruction of neurons and connections infants inter-neurons, similar changes were observed in poisoning with mercury, lead and alcohol. (Waly 2004).

- With each re-vaccination increases the possibility of such local reactions (Werner 1987). At first re-vaccination of students from Sweden, performed at age 10, have been observed with 73% of them local. (Blennow 1984);

- The first day after vaccination, infants have a state of agitation and crying, accompanied by fever, older children accused a general altered slightly, with nausea and headache;

Allergies:

- _Chronic urticarial_ and _asthma symptoms_ occur in 1 in 100,000 cases;

- Allergic shock is rare, but can be deadly;

- 2 weeks after the vaccine may occur _glomerulonephritis_ (kidney disease) (Quast 1997);

- If the vaccine is combined with one or more vaccines (tri- vaccine, tetra- vaccine, penta-vaccine, hexa-6-vaccines), increase the frequency of allergy cases. E.L. Hurwitz (2000) show that the vaccinated children, allergies are twice as common by the age of 16 years, compared with non-vaccinated children;

- How it can cause allergic reactions after tetanus vaccine was described by Italian immunologist Adriano Mari as follows: after the vaccine, the body produces antibodies not only against tetanus toxin, but also against the mast cell-related immunological components, receptors for IgE (Immunological globuline E). As a result, there will be elimination of mediators from mast cells that can cause _allergic reactions such as allergic dermatitis and autoimmune diseases._ (Ibid., p 148-149). "We consider that the tetanus vaccine has greatly contributed to increase the frequency of allergic diseases in the last 30-40 years through its widespread worldwide," said author (Mari 2004);

Thrombocytopenia It is a complication of vaccine, characterized by blood clotting disorders that require medical supervision and treatment.

Myocarditis Is a serious complication, especially in infants, which may cause death (Shye - Jao 2006).

Neurological Most commonly affected nerves are at hand: the brachial plexus or median nerve, resulting in _paralysis of the hand_ (sometimes permanent) _or sensitivity problems, accompanied by sharp pain._ (HRSA 1997, Read 1992, Topaloglu 1992, Pollard 1978, Schlenska 1977);

What "the hell" is swine flu?

- New type of **influenza A H1N1** is unlike any other virus the previous isolation.

- The virus **was synthesized in the laboratory:** Dr. Johan Hultin from Iowa State University, has successfully extracted genetic material from a body fat of 30-something, female, who died of **flu Spanish in 1918,** with 85% of villagers in Brevig Mission (called Teller Mission in 1918), in one week. Victims of Spanish flu that has been extracted genetic material was buried in the Arctic permafrost. This pandemic **killed at least 50 million people worldwide.**

- Scientists have recreated the genetic material of the 1918 Spanish flu virus in a laboratory FINAT U.S. Government. The virus **obtained was then mixed together artificially H3N2 virus and a minor gene splice in Eurasia - H5N1 - avian flu strain.** Or H5N1 bird flu virus that hit Asia in 2006, contains some genetic mutations of the virus in 1918 .

- Finally, this virus contains **genetic material from two strains of swine flu, two strains of human flu and one strain of avian flu;**

   –   - Centres for Disease Control (CDC) called the resulting virus ***"novel flu"***, incorrectly said "swine flu". The current strain of flu *"novel"* is changing rapidly in humans, animals do not "catch" the virus. (Because of the rapid mutations of the virus and the fact that, unlike 1918, now global transport are faster, is normal that scientists estimate that both the molecular clock of A/H1N1 virus and modern means of transport, will make almost all countries in the world have experienced an H1N1 outbreak in the next few months.

   –   What's different about H1N1 virus is that, unlike other new strains of viruses that mutate developing fast, then slow mutations, and finally stopped completely, *"the novel"* yet give no signs of slowing down the rate of mutation, as such, scientists are concerned because H1N1 is not generated synthetically acts as a natural one. ***(Wayne Madsen Report - May 21, 2009.*** *Wayne Madsen is an investigative journalist in Washington DC).*

The viruses are classified by subtype on the basis of two major surface special proteins: hema- glutinin (H) and neuro - aminidase (N). By segmenting the genome, the virus has the ability to rearrange and genomic segments and to recombine, thus increasing the rate of evolution and generation of new strains.

Recombination is widely used in the laboratory to create new vaccines (you may read as ""**new attacks to the immune system of children!!!**"").

SOURCES : Olsen B, Munster VJ, Wallensten A, Waldenstrom J, Osterhaus and Fouchier RAM. Global patterns of influenza A virus in wild birds. Science 2006, 312, 384-8.)

How serious is swine flu?

- **Symptoms of swine flu are at most moderate;**

- In **July 2009** were recorded 40,617 cases of flu in the U.S. of which 319 deaths, which means **a mortality of 0.8%,** although it seems that the death rate was actually much lower. Experts estimate that in fact only one of 20 cases of flu are reported. (2009 flu pandemic in the United States ", Wikipedia, 22 July 2009)

Why are disputed principles of vaccination?

- Flu vaccines are traditionally produced from non-virulent viruses (attenuated or weakened). To be effective vaccines should contain virus affecting the population, but non-virulent form. <u>Vaccine that works by the immune system is activated by exposure to the non-virulent (non-pathogenic) virus and produce antibodies following protect the body against pathogenic form of the virus.</u> *(Hood, 2006, Environmental Health Innovations Perspectives 114, A108-111.)*

— - Recent studies, and older showed that injection of foreign genetic material directly into the bloodstream leading to genetic mutations and cancer genesis (cancer formation) in the body that receives material. Swiss researchers Phillipe Anker and Maurice Stroun at the Laboratory of Biochemistry and Plant Physiology, University of Geneva, pioneers of molecular biology, have regularly published their findings in medical journals continuously from the 60s until now. They have discovered that biological substances entering directly into the bloodstream could become part of the human genetic code.

— Their studies have shown that nucleic acids DNA and RNA in the cell nucleus not only exist, but small amounts of genetic material flow freely into the extracellular space of all living organisms. Most vaccines are made from dormant live viruses.

— **Human cells currently used in vaccine production are so-called cell lines "immortal".** **They are, in fact, cancer cells from different types of human tumours and foetal tissue from aborted human embryos, capable only survive in vitro and divide without limit of time and space.**

— **These cell cultures are fed usually with a nutrient mixture based extract of foetal calf serum. Viruses from vaccines are able to include genetic material in cells that are grown and the nutrient applied, so all ingredients are used in industrial production of vaccines are all sources of contamination of the final product. Purification of total final vaccine is practically impossible, because no laboratory in the world is capable, at present, to separate the entire remaining vaccine virus from the culture medium.**

— **This is officially recognized in that current standards for acceptable contamination considered as vaccine production to 100 pg (pico grammes) of DNA per dose of vaccine.**

— **Now, we know that cancer induction is a phenomenon that starts from a single cell as a single functional unit of foreign DNA into host cell genome can induce malignant cell transformation. In 1960, the SV40 virus (Simian Virus 40) in oral polio vaccine "Sabin", prepared with live virus. It was subsequently discovered that polio vaccine "Salk" (version with inactivated virus, administered by injection) is contaminated, because the virus survives formaldehyde used for inactivation.**

— **Researchers as Sweet and Hilleman of the Merck Institute for**

Therapeutic Research, which made the discovery, said that <u>all three strains of polio vaccine were found infested.</u> SV 40 virus derived from green monkey kidney in Africa, which has grown, always, polio vaccine. Confirmation of the oncogene role of this virus came when the SV40 viral genome was found in various malignant tumours of adults injected with polio vaccine in infancy: *lymphoma, non-Hodgkin's lymphoma , brain tumours, cancer, tumours, etc."*

The hidden viruses, as they were called, have a feature that explains their names while creating destruction marked in vitro and in vivo, they are not recognized by human immune system, because their structure does not have critical antigens necessary for identification. They determine, **therefore, serious illness, train, central and peripheral nervous system, often with fatal outcomes.** Researcher said he found that they can be considered **"a biological weapon of nature",** because they can wear different structural forms, but retains the ability to include the nerve cell and destroy it.

- **- Vaccine Act must be understood ultimately as an act of introducing foreign genetic material directly into the bloodstream.**

- **Mass vaccination campaigns have had an overwhelming impact on the population,** in that it led the long term, the genetic mutations unpredictable and negatively alter the human genetic code.

- **Link between genetic mutations and oncogenes in humans** has been proven scientifically, and increased incidence and mortality from cancer is a reality today.

WHO and fever mass vaccination

Order mass vaccination this fall came from the WHO (World Health Organization). In early July 2009, a group of experts in vaccines concluded that the outbreak is unstoppable and Marie-Paul Kieny, WHO director of vaccine research direction said that all nations will have access to vaccines and the vaccine will be ready for administration in **September.** The "vaccines experts" are influenced by vaccine manufacturers who want to earn huge profits from government contracts.

But the decisive argument against mass vaccination is **that the vaccine is not effective, moreover, is very dangerous.**

- **Professor Dr.Vasile Astarastoae (President of the Medical College of**

Romania): "W.H.O. introduces medical dictatorship! WHO, so far, any assessment would make total proved ineffective. None of WHO programs have failed as they were presented. "In addition, all this escalated alert level was done without the consent of health ministers of member countries OMSOMS is now a" kolhoz "internationally: in the last 25 years, has turned into an institution that maintains its own bureaucracy - as the European Union that goes down the same path. The WHO takes measures to survive. All deaths in the world due to swine flu were people who had already immune-compromised by their previous illness.

- **WHO is trying to introduce a medical dictatorship, as public health (DPH), which began to violate the natural rights of man,** because, see: introduced quarantine prohibited the free **movement, introduced compulsory vaccination, patient autonomy has been violated cannot refuse treatment required.** All on this principle of the community safety. There is a balance between patient rights and the principle of safety. Then enter the WHO, I think it's correct term medical dictatorship.

- We learn, for example, how to eat, without considering that there was a natural selection based on eating behaviour. In addition, at present, **we are making fetishism regarding some concepts in medicine, which again introduce the dictatorship,** such as, for example, guidelines, protocols and evidence-based medicine. ". *(source : no. 6 / 2009 Magazine" Orthodox Press ": Influenza A H1N1 - A PROPAGANDA FOR WHO?).*

The Austrian journalist Jane Burgermeister said that : "Senior U.N. and U.S. officials and W.H.O. are part of an" international crime syndicate "and controlled by bankers managing the Federal Reserve of USA money". (AFTER this declaration she lost her job...).

This group is about to commit "the largest biological genocide" in the world, using the vaccine against the H1N1 virus.

Moreover, it intends to request the prohibition measures forced vaccination of the population in the U.S. and other countries affected by swine flu.

The reporter, the group released an artificially created virus to remove part of the population and to obtain profits from vaccine sales by pharmaceutical companies. In April 2009 she brought out evidence of Baxter Laboratories intentionally released 72 pounds of active avian influenza virus. It seems that the virus was delivered already to WHO by 16 laboratories in four countries. *(In which countries? they did not said.)*

Vaccination at all costs?

 Virus had the flu spreads and, regardless of origin or benign form of flu, which the public are especially worried about the government mass vaccination programs designed to combat the epidemic and that could be worse than the epidemic itself. Thus the U.S. Department of Health and that of National Security said in April shortly after the appearance of epidemic as swine flu is a health emergency.

As a result, some schools were closed, some people put in quarantine and pharmaceutical companies have signed contracts worth a total $ 7 billion to produce vaccines that will be circulated by the Food and Drug Administration.

This means that vaccines will be tested for only a few weeks to hundreds of volunteers: children and adults before being administered to all pupils, in autumn 2009, starting in October.

Moreover, as a result of federal legislation adopted by Congress in 2001, an authorization for emergency use permit pharmaceutical companies, health system officials and anyone who deals with experimental vaccines that during a state of emergency, are protected legal if the population suffer injuries following vaccination.

Health and Human Services Secretary Kathleen Sebelius, has provided manufacturers of vaccines, total immunity before the law, against any claim in court that could result from vaccination.

Some states want to impose compulsory vaccination *law.*

(*Http://* www.isis.org.uk/fastTrackSwineFluVaccineUnderFire.php).

a) *the vaccine is dangerous*

- Vaccine itself can be dangerous, especially **germ attenuated** vaccines or **new vaccines recombinant nucleic acids** (as in the case of swine flu), they having a potential to generate virulent strains through recombination and the recombinant nucleic acids can cause autoimmune diseases.

- — - **Increases the risk of asthma:** a study of 800 children with asthma showed that those who have been vaccinated against influenza have conducted a large number of doctor visits in the emergency room because of problems caused by asthma.

- — This study was supported by a report in 2009 showing that children with asthma who were vaccinated with influenza vaccine had a three times higher risk of hospitalization;

- **Guillain-Barre syndrome:** *is an autoimmune disease that causes paralysis of the arms and legs and, in rare cases, the entire body.* In some cases, GBS but led to complete paralysis or even death;

- — **A major source of toxicity is the flu vaccine adjutants,** substances that are meant to amplify the action of vaccines: Most vaccines have dangerously high mercury content in the form of **thimerosal** *(Preservative lethal) 50 times more toxic than mercury itself.* A large enough dose can cause dysfunction at long-term immune, sensory, neurological, motor and behavioural.

Mercury poisoning leading to autism, attention deficient syndrome, Multiple sclerosis, speech and language impairments. Another common adjutant is aluminium hydroxide vaccines causing allergy and anaphylaxis. Most new adjutants, including *MF59, ISCOMS, OS21, AS02 and AS04* are more toxic than aluminium hydroxide. . 40-42, 2007.) Some doses of vaccine will contain **squalene** *causing Gulf War syndrome and other disabilities. (How to stop tax INSTEAD of the flu vaccine-antiviral model. (Science in Society 35 . 40-42, 2007.)*

b) the vaccine is ineffective

Numerous studies show that anti-influenza vaccine protects little or nothing and there is reason to believe that swine flu vaccine will be different; The prevention of other influenza-illness was only 33-36%. ; *(Swine flu pandemic now 'Unstoppable': WHO official ", Agence France-Presse, 13 July 2009, Calgary Herald, http://www.calgaryherald.com /Swine+pandemic+unstoppable+official/1788693/story.html).*

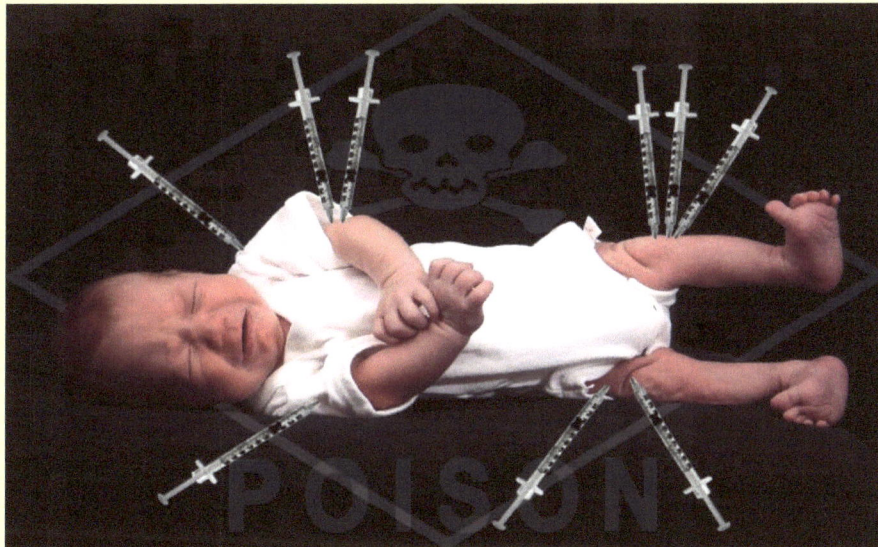

The greatest LIE ever old is that vaccines are safe and effective" -

DR.L.HOROWITZ

A few words about

who makes the vaccines

Everyone knows that 5 big companies have global contracts to produce vaccines: Baxter International,   Glaxo-SmithKline, Novartis, Aventis , Sanofis -AstroZeneca.

What are these companies?

a) Novartis has caused a media scandal in 2008 as a result of clinical trials with H5N1 (avian influenza) held in Poland. Testing consisted of administering the vaccine to 350 homeless by Polish nurses and doctors, which led to the deaths of 21 of the test and bringing the medical staff in court by the Polish police. Novartis claimed at the time the deaths were not caused by the vaccine they also said "3500 was tested without problems on other people".

Also Novartis announced June 13 that the swine flu vaccine produced using all technology based on cell culture and adjutant MF59. This adjutant is oily nature and contains Tween80, Span85 and squalene. Studies in mice have shown that oily adjutants induce motor problems and paralysis. Squalene induces severe arthritis in mice and in human subjects found that administration of squalene between 10 and 20 ppm (parts per billion) lead to serious system problems immune and autoimmune diseases occurrence.;

b) France ordered vaccines from Sanofi, GSK and Novartis, but sees no reason why clinical trials should be shortened. French pharmaceutical company Sanofi-Aventis

100

is developing its own vaccine against swine flu will test you in early August. It is estimated that it will take two months and a half of testing for a vaccine to obtain "effective and safe" as Albert Garcia shows company spokesman also said that "the vaccine will be ready in November or December". (Update: January-Baxter CAN take no more H1N1 flu vaccine orders ", Bill Berkerto, 16 July 2009, Reuters.)

c) vaccine from GlaxoSmithKline (GSK) will be produced from antigens insulation recent influenza strains and will contain adjutant AS03 which was approved by the EU with H5N1 bird flu vaccine in 2008. Under the European Public Assessment AS03 contains the poison named squalene (10.68 milligrams), DL-alpha-tocopherol (11.86 milligrams) and polysorbate 80 (4.85 milligrams). H5N1 vaccine also contains 5 milligrams thiomersal (mercury derivative), polysorbate 80, octoxynol 10 and various inorganic salts.

The company aggressively are promoting various adjutant systems as the "adjutant advantageous" to reduce the dose of vaccine. GSK vaccines it will be tested on a small number of people while the company reportedly looking to "weigh the danger of pandemic vaccine against the risks of potentially dangerous".

 This was characterized as risky by **Professor Hugh Pennington**, a retired microbiologist at **Aberdeen University, Scotland**. *"By limiting clinical trials, Glaxo risks not calibrate the optimal dose of the vaccine and this would lead to a vaccination not only protects Worse population puts health at risk"* showed DR. Pennington.

 d) Baxter instead has begun In December 2008. A subsidiary company of Baxter in Austria sent for testing human flu vaccines contaminated with the lethal strain of avian influenza H5N1 virus in 18 countries including Czech Republic, where tests were killed laboratory animals used. At that time, Czech newspapers questioned if company Baxter deliberately tried to stir a pandemic to make huge money as profit from sold out vaccines on market. (http://infowars.net /articles /august2009/100809Czech.htm).

The Genetically Modified Viruses

Genetically modified (GM) vaccines are already being produced and we know very little about their long-term effects and nobody knows well what happens when children and people are receiving this kind of vaccines.

There have been some fair warnings, though. In 2006, researchers wrote in the Journal of Toxicology and Environmental Health: "Genetically modified (GM) viruses and genetically engineered virus-vector vaccines possess significant unpredictability and a number of inherent harmful potential hazards… Horizontal transfer of genes… is well established. New hybrid

101

virus progenies resulting from genetic recombination between genetically engineered vaccine viruses and their naturally occurring relatives may possess totally unpredictable characteristics with regard to host preferences and disease-causing potentials.

...There is inadequate knowledge to define either the probability of unintended events or the consequences of genetic modifications."

Though this was six years ago, little has changed even as the technology has advanced. Today we have several different types of GM vaccines in production, development or research phases, such as:

DNA vaccines: DNA for a microbe's antigens are introduced into the body, with the expectation that your cells will take up that DNA, which then instructs your cells to make antigen molecules.

As the National Institute of Allergy and Infectious Disease (a division of the National Institutes of Health) put it, "In other words, the body's own cells become vaccine-making factories."

-Naked DNA vaccines: A type of DNA vaccine in which microscopic particles coated with DNA are administered directly into your cells.

-Recombinant Vector vaccines: Similar to DNA vaccines, but they use a virus or bacteria to act as a vector (or "carrier) to introduce microbial DNA into your cells.

Use of foreign DNA in various forms has the potential to cause a great deal of trouble, not only because there is the potential for it to recombine with our own DNA, but also there is the potential for it to turn the DNA "switches," the epigenetic parts of the DNA, on and off

GM vaccines are already in use and are being administered to American infants, children and adults. This has been going on for many years.

Hepatitis B vaccine: An inactivated recombinant DNA vaccine licensed for newborn infants and children in 1991, in which parts of the hepatitis B virus gene are cloned into yeast

Rota-virus vaccine: Live attenuated vaccines first licensed for infants and children licensed in 2006, which either contain genetically engineered human rota-virus strains or human-bovine hybridized re assortment rota virus strains.

HPV vaccine (Gardasil or Cervarix): A recombinant vaccine licensed in 2006, which is prepared from virus-like particles (VLP's) and may also include use of an insect-cell Baculovirus expression vector system for production of vaccines.

Most vaccine revenues are earned by five companies that together held nearly 80 percent of the market in 2010:

Sanofi Pasteur

Glaxo Smith Kline

Merck & Co.

Pfizer and Novartis.

These five very big companies, which use genetic engineering to produce vaccines, are also primarily responsible for the introduction of genetic engineering into the food supply.

In fact, they went to work for U.S. corporations and pharmaceutical companies that run the vaccine industry today.

At least a dozen of these cold blooded killers were hired fresh out of prison, just 4 to 7 years after the Nuremberg trials found them guilty of mass murder and enslavement.

Herr S Carl Krauch, Executive Member of IG Farben and Head of Military Economics for Hitler, found guilty of slavery and mass murder, served just 6 years in prison, then became Chairman of the Board for BASF in 1952.

This is the same vaccine industry today which protected and employed Nazi war criminals. The industry that produced the Nazi gas chambers was purchased by Bayer.

So, exactly whom are you trusting with your children's health and welfare?

Do you want more research before you or your children get injected with a new concocted disease for which there is no cure? Listen to stunning admissions by vaccine industry experts, including Dr. Maurice Hilleman (formerly /Merck), who admitted to the deadly nature of the most trusted vaccines. (source http://tv.naturalnews.com/v.asp?v=13EAAF22CDA367BB3C2F94D2CD90EF7B)

MY CONCLUSIONS

The MEDICINE UNIVERSITIES all over the world SHOULD CHANGE COMPULSORY THE "TABU" IDEAS OF VACCINATIONS.

The vaccines are useless and very dangerous for health and contains POISONS. When a doctor is learning in the medicine school about what good is the vaccine, at that time were not health studies about LONG-TERM EFFECTS OF VACCINES.

DO NOT TRUST YOUR DOCTOR 100% ! Do not be trustworthy blind!

ASK QUESTIONS ABOUT VACCINES AND ASK ABOUT HIS SIGNATURE !

IF HE RECOMMENDS VACCINES TO YOU AND YOUR CHILDREN, YOUR DOCTOR HAS TO SIGN A PAPER ABOUT POSSIBLE SIDE-EFFECTS AND THAT HE WILL PAY BIG MONEY TO YOUR FAMILY IF VACCINES DO NOT WORK. *Do you know that your doctor will never sign that paper?*

Today we have this studies and medical proofs that vaccines are not good for health. Soon will be another pathology to be written, for vaccinated society, a weak society with the immune system devastated and DNA changed after generations of immunization campaigns.

The pharmaceutical industries are making hundreds of billions of dollars, Euro and GBP and the vaccinated society is their faithfully client. The vaccines can kill children and that vaccinated children lost their health for ever!

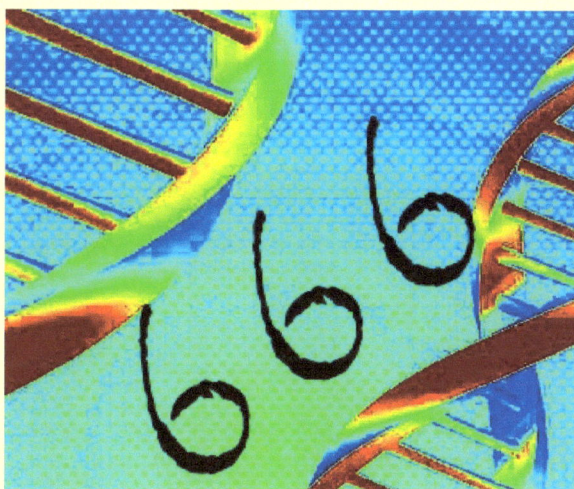

The biggest mistake in your life is to accept that the vaccines are miracles! The vaccines are useless and very dangerous for health.

Writing about the dangers of vaccination, I know that this is a concept that you find difficult to accept by stubborn people. However, today (end of the year 2013) it is at stake your health and yours children's health...

GOD made perfect the human body.

*If you forget GOD, **tomorrow** will come the alternative evil 666 in your life!*

Say NO to vaccines!

May GOD help YOU!

28th of December 2013

www.ingramcontent.com/pod-product-compliance
Lightning Source LLC
Chambersburg PA
CBHW041720210326
41598CB00007B/721